SLOW
COOKING

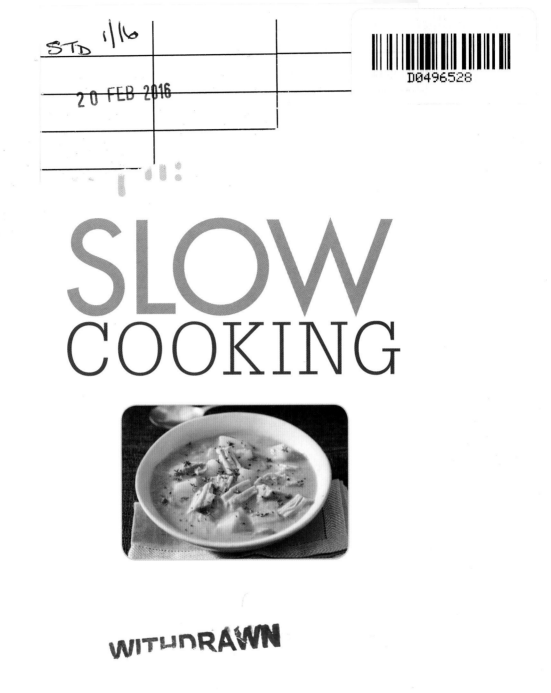

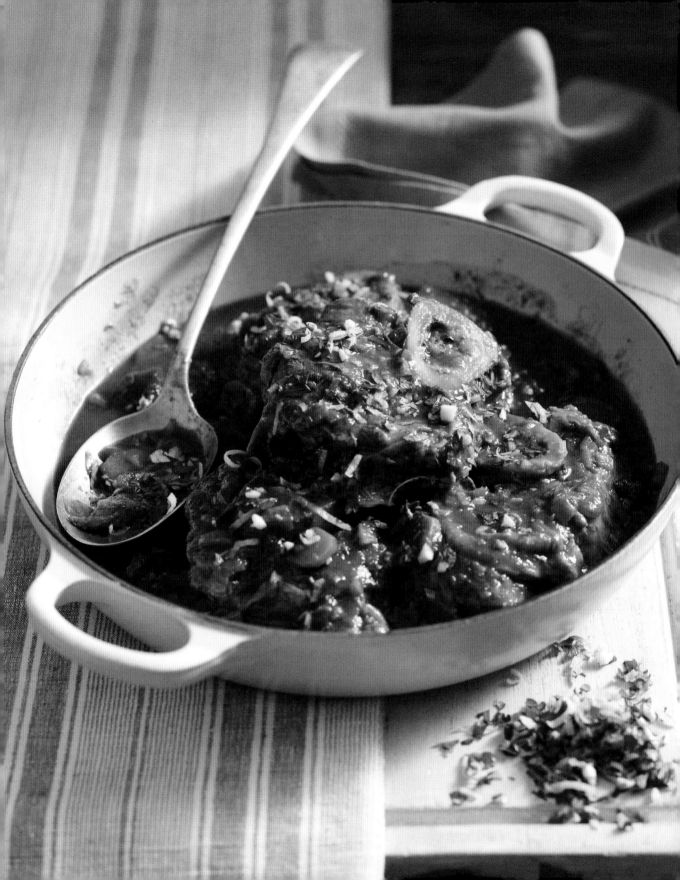

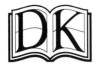

try it!

SLOW
COOKING

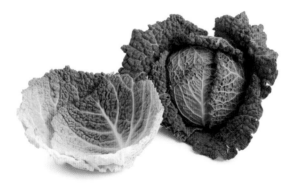

HEATHER WHINNEY

Penguin Random House

Photography Stuart West
Recipe Editor Emma Callery

DK UK

Project Editor Kathryn Meeker
Senior Art Editor Anne Fisher
Managing Editor Stephanie Farrow
Managing Art Editor Christine Keilty
Jacket Designer Amy Keast
Producer, Pre-Production Andy Hilliard
Producer Stephanie McConnell
Art Director Maxine Pedliham
Publisher Mary-Clare Jerram

DK INDIA

Project Editor Arani Sinha
Senior Art Editor Ivy Roy
Art Editor Jomin Johny
Deputy Managing Editor Bushra Ahmed
Managing Art Editor Navidita Thapa
Pre-Production Manager Sunil Sharma
Senior DTP Designer Pushpak Tyagi
DTP Designer Manish Upreti

First published in Great Britain in 2016 by
Dorling Kindersley Limited,
80 Strand, London WC2R 0RL

Copyright © 2016 Dorling Kindersley Limited
A Penguin Random House Company
2 4 6 8 10 9 7 5 3 1
001 – 289129– Jan/2016

A CIP catalogue record for this book
is available from the British Library.
ISBN 978-0-2412-4073-1

Printed and bound in China.

All images © Dorling Kindersley Limited
For further information see: www.dkimages.com

A WORLD OF IDEAS:
SEE ALL THERE IS TO KNOW

www.dk.com

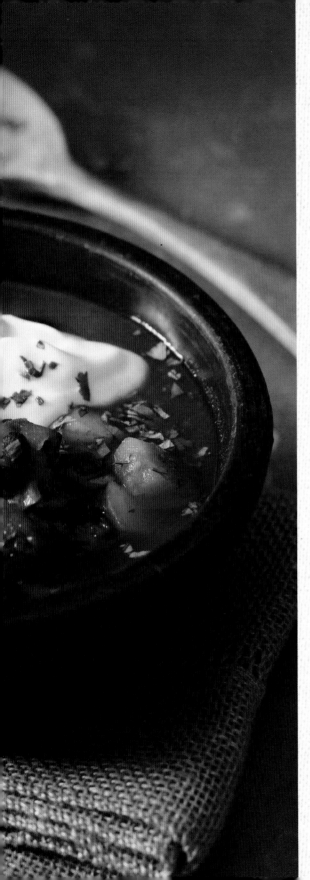

Contents

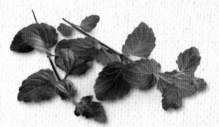

Note:
All the recipes in this book are written for the medium size range of slow cookers, from a minimum of 3.5 litres to 5 litres capacity. Allowances should be made for the differences within this size range; depending on the internal volume of your slow cooker, liquid quantities may need to be adjusted to ensure the food is covered where necessary.

Foreword

I am generally not a fan of kitchen gadgets, but I have to admit to being a convert to the slow cooker. The thrifty cook in me is thoroughly excited by using the cheaper cuts of meat and beans and pulses that are so suited to slow cooking, while the ease of throwing a collection of ingredients into a pot and letting them do their own thing for hours is enormously attractive – so little effort is needed, but the rewards are great.

Our attitude towards food and cooking is changing. We seem to have a stronger desire to make home-cooked food that nourishes us and our family, as well as reining in our spending. Slow cooking is perfect for meeting this need – it suits every level of cook, especially the novice, as it is a style of cooking that doesn't rely heavily on precision. It's one of the most forgiving cooking techniques, requiring little time or skill from the cook. Moreover, by its very nature, slow cooking isn't an extravagant way to cook. By choosing value cuts and seasonal produce we naturally spend less, and the running costs of a slow cooker are minimal, little more than running a low watt light bulb, consequently conserving energy.

The great benefits of the slow cooker lie in its convenience and versatility. To be able to simply "set and forget" the slow cooker has enormous advantages for our hectic lives – it can sit day or night unattended. It ticks all the boxes for such a wide range of people: those cooking for one, large families, busy mums, and it's ideal for entertaining as it makes dinner party cooking a breeze. I didn't at first realise the potential of the slow cooker; as well as casseroles and stews, it can be used to cook whole joints of meat, delicate risottos, and delicious soups. It can also be used as a water bath or bain-marie for puddings and desserts.

The practical nature of slow cooking greatly appeals to me. It lends itself to cooking in large batches, and I love being able to cook up something delicious to serve one day and perhaps freeze for another. It is extremely satisfying to know there is the option of leftovers, thus relieving that sometimes niggling pressure of knowing what we are going to cook for dinner the next night. Of course it requires some planning, as does all cooking, but through this it also reduces food waste, which I feel passionately about. Again, the thrifty cook in me rearing its head!

Although we always think of simmering pots of meat and vegetables when slow cooking is mentioned, I think it is fair to say that the slow cooker isn't just for cold winter days. In fact, it is ideal in summer, for maybe a curry or ribs, when you don't want the heat of the cooker on all day. I've tried to reflect this throughout the book so you can always find inspiration as you dip in and out throughout the seasons.

This book contains more than 80 recipes for slow cooking. It includes a mixture of world cuisines, features many classics, and offers some new adventurous flavour combinations. Chapters cover Soups and Broths; Stews; Casseroles and Cassoulets; Tagines; Curries; Chillies and Gumbos; Pot Roasts and Ribs; Risottos, Pilafs, and Paellas; and a Puddings chapter that includes favourites such as crème caramel.

Step-by-step photographs take you through the types of slow cooking, from stewing to poaching, as well as the principles of slow cooking, such as browning ingredients and reducing sauces. A comprehensive list is also given for the slow cook's storecupboard, as a well-stocked larder is a great asset; once you have this, you need shop for little else but the perishables.

I hope this book inspires you to experiment with slow cooking. Let your imagination conjure up the thought of boeuf bourguignon, the beef nestling in a mixture of heady red wine and robust herbs, cooked to perfection until it melts in your mouth; or a slow-cooked pork dish such as belly pork and prunes cooked with earthy celeriac and sage, and simmered slowly in a little wine until the pork falls apart at the touch of your fork. Just the thought of it makes you want to head off into the kitchen and reach for your apron!

Heather Whinney

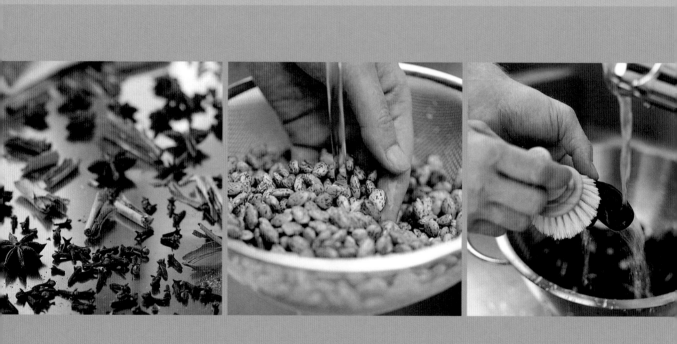

Techniques

Slow cooking is ideal for many households, from the time-poor cook's to the frugal one's. Food can be left unattended, less expensive ingredients can be used, and it delivers a nutritious meal at the end of the day.

Why slow cook?

Slow cooking is a method of cooking food slowly, as the name suggests, but not all food that is cooked slowly can be defined as "slow cook". To "slow cook" means that ingredients are cooked for a long time at a low heat, in a cooking pot with a fitted lid, and either covered or partially covered in liquid. Stews, casseroles, and pot roasts are all examples of slow cook dishes, and all are satisfyingly simple to make.

Prep and forget

Any cooking involves a certain amount of preparation, but with slow cooking this is kept to a minimum, as practically all the labour takes place early on in the cooking process. Once the food is in the cooking pot, it can be left to its own devices, requiring minimal attention from you. However, planning your meals and organizing your shopping list is essential – it will enable you to assemble a dish effortlessly.

Maximize flavour

When left to slow cook, ingredients marry together and the flavours intensify. When meat is slow cooked, the gelatine is extracted from the meat and bones, which results in a rich, concentrated sauce; it is this exchange of flavours between the meat and sauce that gives slow cooking its wonderful rich but mellow taste. Aromatic vegetables and spices such as cloves, cinnamon, and star anise are great to use as their distinct flavours are not lost when slow cooked.

Be thrifty

Slow cooking makes economic sense as it works best using cheaper cuts of meat that have high bone and fat content, and inexpensive staples such as beans and lentils. It is also easy to cook large quantities at once, creating leftovers for another day or to freeze. Slow cooking is also an opportunity to be creative and make meals out of very little – long, gentle cooking will turn the remnants of your refrigerator or storecupboard into a feast.

Tips for success

Choosing the right equipment and using your ingredients with a little know-how will help you achieve great results from slow cooking.

For traditional slow cooking, choose a thick-walled flameproof casserole that holds the heat well, such as a cast-iron one or an enamelled cast-iron one. Ensure it has a well fitting lid and can be used on the hob or in the oven. Cast-iron casseroles can be heavy, so choose one with two easy-to-hold handles. Pick a size to suit your requirements: as a rule of thumb, food should only reduce down to about three-quarters of the pot's volume once cooked from full.

Moroccan tagines, cone-shaped earthenware cooking pots with tall lids, are apt for slow cooking. They are designed to return condensation back into the dish to keep the food moist. For versatility, choose one that can be used on the hob (with a diffuser) and the oven.

For maximum flavour, brown the meat at the start of cooking, and soften aromatic vegetables such as onions and garlic by sautéing.

Be careful not to over season; salty flavours become concentrated with slow cooking. Season lightly initially, then adjust at the end of cooking if needed.

Peppercorns and seeds, such as cumin, coriander, and fennel, are best crushed before adding to the pot so they release their flavour slowly.

Woody herbs, such as rosemary and thyme, are robust enough to add at the beginning of cooking; add delicate herbs, such as parsley, towards the end of cooking, or stir into the finished dish.

Always add delicate ingredients that don't need much cooking, such as fish and seafood, towards the end of the cooking time.

If topping up the liquid during cooking, add hot liquid to prevent lowering the cooking temperature.

Clockwise from top left: slow cooking lends itself to soothing soups (Pumpkin and ginger soup p62), fresh and light risottos (Risotto primavera p166), hearty casseroles (Osso bucco p94), and tasty puddings (Apple dumplings p186).

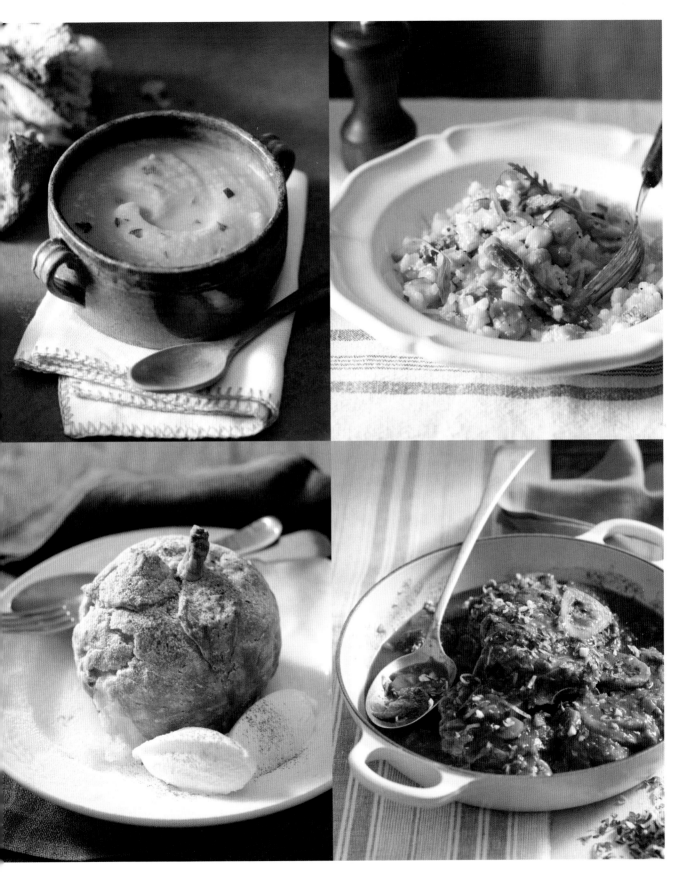

With so many slow cookers on the market it is important that you choose one to suit your needs. There are certain variables, both in terms of design and price, but slow cookers generally operate on similar principles.

How to use your slow cooker

A slow cooker consists of a sturdy, heatproof outer casing and an inner cooking pot into which the food is placed. The outer casing is made of either stainless steel or aluminium and is where the heating element and controls are housed. The inner cooking pot is usually removable. The lid on a slow cooker fits snugly so that heat cannot escape. The condensation that occurs during the slow, low-heat cooking process gathers around the lip of the pot and creates a water seal. The condensation is then released back into the pot and it is this that keeps the food moist. The combination of a long cooking time and the steam that is created within the pot destroys any bacteria, making it a safe cooking method. It is important to resist the temptation to open the lid to look – this will release heat and break the water seal and you will need to add a further 20 minutes to the cooking time.

Choosing the right shape and size

Slow cookers come in a range of sizes, but small machines start from 1.5 litres (2¾ pints), which is suitable for 1–2 people; a medium-sized 3.5-litre (6-pint) cooker is great for 4 people; for 6 people or more, choose a 5-litre (8¾-pint) model or larger. However, bigger isn't necessarily better unless you are catering for large numbers or wish to batch cook – you need to half-fill a slow cooker for optimum performance, and accommodate it on your kitchen worktop, so choose wisely. Slow cookers can be either round or oval in shape; the choice is down to personal preference. Casseroles, chillies, and curries are all perfect for round cookers but an oval one is preferable if you wish to cook whole joints of meat or chickens, and fit in pudding basins or ramekins. The removable inner cooking pots are usually ceramic, but they are also available in cast-aluminium. Ceramic pots are easiest to wash and clean, retain the heat well, and can be served straight to the table. Cast-aluminium pots are lighter and allow you to brown food in them first before cooking. Always choose a slow cooker with a recognised safety mark.

Adapting recipes for the slow cooker

You can easily adapt conventional recipes for the slow cooker. Firstly, find a recipe in this book that is similar in style and has similar ingredients, such as the meat cuts, beans, or vegetables. From this you can ascertain the length of cooking time needed. If you are at all worried, leave it to cook for longer – a slow cooker won't boil dry. Secondly, adjust the ingredient quantities to ensure they will all fit in the pot. Finally, as a general guide, halve the liquid in your recipe. This is because the liquid doesn't evaporate in the slow cooker as it does with other methods. You can always top it up if needed, or if you do find yourself with too much, remove the lid and cook on High until the excess liquid has evaporated away. When adapting recipes, bear the following in mind:

The recipe must contain some liquid if going into the slow cooker.

Make sure all frozen ingredients are thawed and meats are thoroughly defrosted before cooking.

If a recipe calls for milk, cream, or soured cream, only add this for the last 30 minutes of cooking. For best results, stir in cream just before serving.

You may need to reduce spices and herbs as their flavour becomes concentrated in the slow cooker.

GENERAL GUIDE TO COOKING TIMES

The table below indicates preferred cooking times, but refer to your manufacturer's instructions.

	Low	High
Meat stews and casseroles	6–8 hours	3–4 hours
Pot roasts	6–8 hours	3–4 hours
Whole chickens	6–8 hours	3–4 hours
Ribs	6–8 hours	n/a
Dried beans	6–8 hours	3–4 hours
Steamed puddings	n/a	3–4 hours

Using the slow cooker

Slow cookers are more efficient than traditional ovens and can help to reduce your fuel bill as they use minimum electricity – often only as much as a low watt light bulb. The vast majority of slow cookers have only 2 or 3 heat settings, making them very easy to use. For best results, the slow cooker should be at least half full but no more than two-thirds full when cooking.

Lid – glass lids allow you to check the food without breaking the water seal.

Inner cooking pot – usually removable to make cleaning easier.

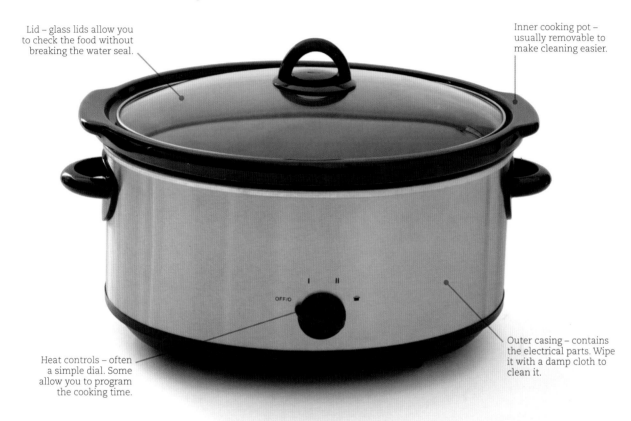

Heat controls – often a simple dial. Some allow you to program the cooking time.

Outer casing – contains the electrical parts. Wipe it with a damp cloth to clean it.

HEAT SETTINGS

The various slow cooker models have different functions for heat settings, but as a rule they all have low and high. Some also have auto, warm, or even medium settings. Preheating the slow cooker before use raises the temperature of the pot before adding the food. The necessity of doing this differs for each slow cooker so it is advisable to read the manufacturer's instructions for your model.

Low: This is the lowest temperature you can cook at and is ideal for leaving food throughout the day or overnight. It is the best setting for cheaper cuts of meat. Cooking times for low vary between 6–12 hours. The food will cook at around 100°C (200°F).

High: This setting is around 150°C (300°F), and in general the food cooks between 3–6 hours. As a rule of thumb, the high setting takes half as long as the low one, so 1 hour on the high setting equals 2 hours on low.

Auto: This setting starts cooking the food on high for 1 hour then reduces it to the low temperature for the remainder of the cooking time.

Keep warm: This holds the food at a lower temperature than low to keep it at an ideal heat for serving. Many cookers switch to this setting automatically once the food is cooked. However, do not leave the food standing in the cooker keeping warm for longer than 1–2 hours.

There are various types of slow cooking methods, which you can do traditionally or in the slow cooker. Poaching involves gentle simmering in water, braising is excellent for sealing in flavour before long cooking, stewing produces wonderful sauces where the ingredients have melded together, and pot roasting is ideal for cooking whole joints of meat.

Types of slow cooking

Poaching

The ingredients are immersed in water, then simmered very gently. This is good for both delicate meats, such as fish or chicken breast, and dense or tough meats, such as silverside of beef; a clean, silky texture is achieved. A fitted lid is essential for keeping the moisture in the pan. Never attempt to rush poaching – hard boiling dries out meat. The traditional method (shown with chicken) is described here, but if using a slow cooker, simplify it by adding the meat, water, and any flavourings to the pot at the beginning.

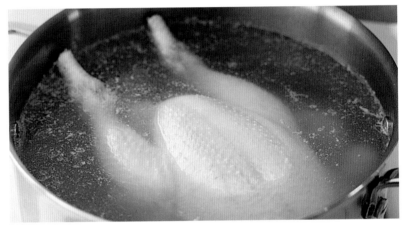

1 Use enough cold water to cover the meat, then bring the water to the boil. Add a pinch of salt and the meat. Reduce the heat and bring back to a gentle simmer, cover the pan with the lid, and poach for 30 minutes.

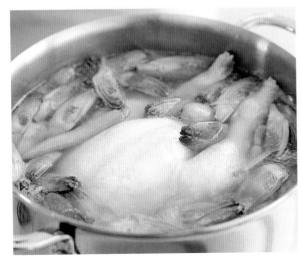

2 Add vegetables to flavour the stock, such as artichokes, carrots, broad beans, and any other green vegetables you want to include – maybe shredded cabbage or runner beans – and cook for 5–10 minutes until they are tender.

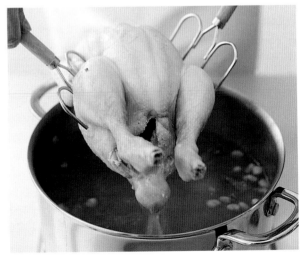

3 To test the chicken for doneness, pierce the thigh to the bone – if the juices run clear it is done, if they are red it is not. Tip the bird slightly as you lift it out of the pan so that the hot stock in its cavity runs back into the pan.

Braising

This technique combines both dry heat and moist heat cooking. The meat, poultry, or vegetables are first seared in hot fat and then cooked slowly in a pan with minimal liquid, just enough to cover. Searing helps to keep the meat succulent. The meat is cut into slightly larger pieces than for stewing. Slightly more expensive cuts can be used for braising, although this technique works just as well with cheap cuts. Braising suits cuts such as brisket, shanks, and oxtail very well. The traditional method steps are shown here, but the process is the same for the slow cooker up to step 3; after the alcohol has evaporated, transfer everything to the slow cooker, pour over the stock, and cook on either setting.

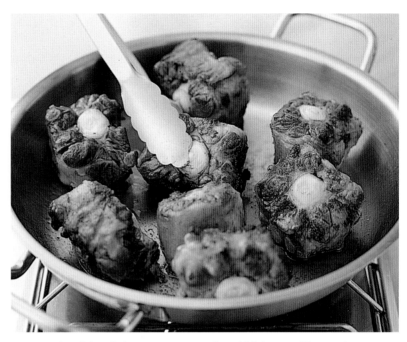

1 Heat the oil in a frying pan over a medium-high heat and brown the meat. Let the pieces sit for about 5 minutes until brown underneath, then turn them and cook the other side for another 5 minutes. Remove with a slotted spoon and set aside.

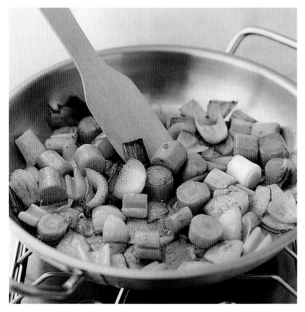

2 Add a mixture of aromatic vegetables, such as carrots, onions, celery, and leeks, stir well with a spatula to collect the meat residue, then cook until the vegetables are browned. Add flavourings, such as thyme, bay leaves, and garlic, and continue to cook for a few minutes more.

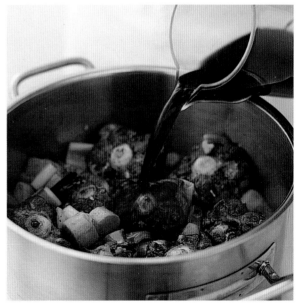

3 Put the meat and vegetables in a flameproof casserole, pour in some wine, and boil over a high heat until nearly evaporated. Add enough stock to cover the meat. Bring to a simmer, cover with the lid, and cook in the oven on a low heat until the meat is tender.

Stewing

Here the ingredients are simmered fully covered in stock or water, and sometimes wine. This is great for tougher cuts as the connective tissue and fat break down while cooking, releasing gelatinous juices and making the meat tender. For a slow cooker, transfer everything to the slow cooker at the end of step 3.

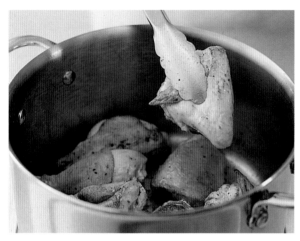

1 Cut the meat into large bite-sized pieces and toss in flour, if you wish (this will help to thicken the stew later). Sear the meat in hot fat and cook for about 5–8 minutes until browned on all sides. Remove and set aside.

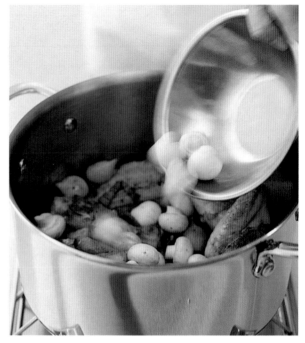

2 Add a selection of vegetables and cook for 5 minutes until golden. Remove and set aside. Deglaze the pan with a little stock or wine and return the meat and vegetables with any sturdy herbs, such as rosemary.

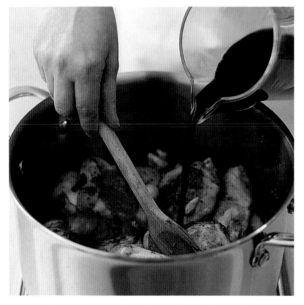

3 Pour in any remaining wine and enough stock to cover the contents of the pan completely. Raise the heat and bring to the boil.

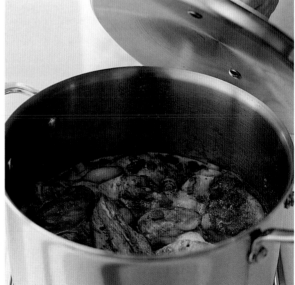

4 Reduce the heat to bring to a gentle simmer and cover with the lid. Cook in the oven on a low heat for a few hours, until the meat is tender.

Pot roasting

This is essentially a braised dish that uses a whole joint of meat, usually of a tougher cut. Liquid is used to barely cover the meat, and vegetables and herbs are added to the pot. A pot roast is cooked in a covered pot on a low heat in the oven or slow cooker for several hours, until the meat is fork tender. The whole joint is usually browned first as this improves the flavour of the finished dish. If using a slow cooker, transfer everything to the slow cooker at the end of step 2, pour over the stock, and cook on auto/low.

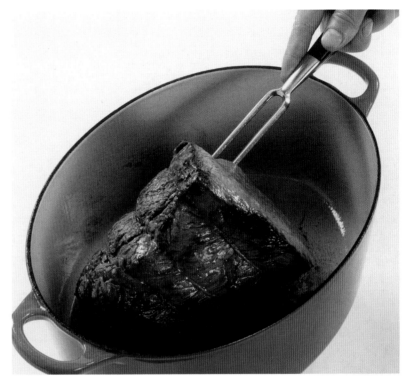

1 Heat 2 tbsp of oil in a flameproof casserole until very hot. Add the meat (it should sizzle) and brown it well on all sides. Remove the casserole from the heat, take out the meat, and discard all but 2 tbsp of fat from the casserole.

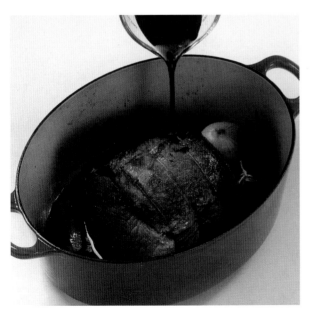

2 Return the meat to the casserole and add vegetables and herbs of your choice. Pour in some wine and cook on the hob for a few minutes so that the alcohol evaporates.

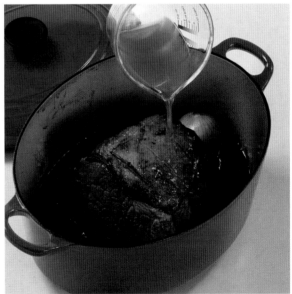

3 Pour in the stock and stir well. Cook for about 3 hours in a low oven, turning the meat 3 or 4 times, and topping up with more stock if too much liquid evaporates.

Keeping a good storecupboard makes any style of cooking easier, but it can really come into its own if you are slow cooking. It reduces the need to plan too far ahead so you can cook spontaneously and decrease your shopping trips. The storecupboard shouldn't be just a place to keep half-open packs and half-used jars; when it is organized well with staple ingredients, you can create meals with only a few fresh additions.

The slow cooking storecupboard

Flavourings

Pastes, seasonings, and oils contribute vital flavour – a spoonful of Thai curry paste or a dab of French mustard can determine the cuisine of your dish in an instant. Use honeys to adjust the sweetness of a marinade. Both olive oil and sunflower oil are versatile enough to be used at high and low temperatures.

- Tomato purée
- Thai curry paste – red and green
- Assorted mustards
- Black peppercorns – whole and crushed
- Sea salt
- Honey
- Olive oil
- Sunflower oil

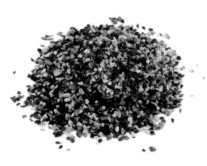

Crushed black peppercorns

Canned and jarred ingredients

An assortment of cans and jars is indispensible for slow cooking. Tomatoes form the base of many stews and ragù dishes, while coconut milk is useful for curries and soups. Choose full-fat varieties of coconut milk though, as low-fat versions can split on cooking. Canned sweetcorn and jarred olives are a great way to add vegetables when you have none in the fridge.

- Tomatoes
- Sun-dried tomatoes
- Coconut milk
- Dried mushrooms
- Anchovies
- Sweetcorn
- Pulses
- Olives
- Capers

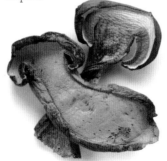

Dried mushrooms

Grains and pasta

Store a range of pasta shapes and sizes so you can add them to soups or casseroles. They are good for late additions to the pot or to serve as accompaniments, as are noodles. Grains such as rice, pearl barley, or farro will happily simmer slowly on a low heat.

- Rice – basmati, white, and brown
- Risotto rice – arborio or carnaroli
- Pearl barley and farro
- Dried pasta
- Dried noodles – rice and egg

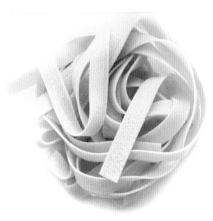

Dried pasta

Sauces and stocks

A good selection of sauces and stocks gives you countless options. Use sauces for marinades or for adjusting flavour at the end of cooking. Vinegars can be used to deglaze after browning, adding richness and depth to your dish. While fresh stock is preferable, powdered stock, or bouillon, is an essential item to keep in the storecupboard if you like to cook without planning too far ahead. Be careful with seasoning, however, when you use powdered stocks – they often contain added salt, so taste your dish first before adding any extra seasoning.

- Soy sauce
- Fish sauce
- Tabasco sauce
- Worcestershire sauce
- Flavoured vinegars – white wine, red wine, and cider
- Balsamic vinegar
- Rice wine vinegar
- Powdered stock (bouillon) – vegetable, chicken, and beef

Beans and pulses

All beans and pulses are ideal for slow cooking. They retain their shape and texture if cooked for a long time and they are a good way of adding bulk and protein to a dish. They also keep indefinitely, so there is no fear of them spoiling. Plan ahead, as most pulses need soaking overnight, except lentils, which just need rinsing well. The older the pulses, the longer they will need soaking.

- Kidney beans
- Cannellini beans
- Haricot beans
- Butterbeans
- Black beans
- Black-eyed beans
- Adzuki beans
- Borlotti beans
- Flageolet beans
- Pinto beans
- Chickpeas
- Yellow and green split peas
- Red lentils
- Puy lentils

Spices and dried herbs

Herbs and spices play an important role in slow cooking, especially if cooking cheaper cuts of meat, as they can transform a simple dish into something special. It is always advisable to taste at the end of cooking and adjust herbs and spices as necessary.

- Allspice
- Cinnamon – ground and sticks
- Coriander seeds
- Cumin – ground and seeds
- Caraway seeds
- Cardamom pods
- Chilli flakes
- Cayenne pepper
- Cloves – ground
- Curry powder
- Fennel seeds
- Ginger – ground
- Juniper berries
- Mustard seeds
- Nutmeg – whole
- Paprika
- Saffron threads
- Star anise
- Turmeric
- Dried oregano

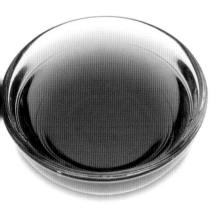

Red wine vinegar

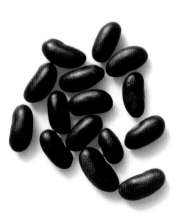

Kidney beans

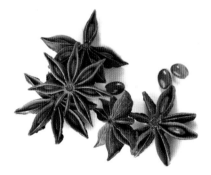

Star anise

As with any cooking, good ingredients will produce good results, but this doesn't necessarily mean choosing expensive ingredients. Slow cooking enables you to make the best possible food with whatever is available, whether it's a collection of humble root vegetables, a cheap meat cut, or some fresh seafood. All it requires is time and care so it can be cooked to perfection.

Choosing and using ingredients

Vegetables

As a rule, the harder, tougher vegetables respond best to slow cooking as it turns them deliciously sweet and tender. The more delicate vegetables should be added to the pot later so they don't fall apart while cooking.

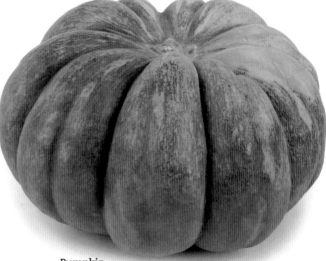

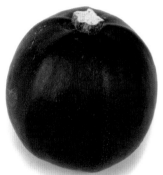

Gem squash
This small squash is sweeter than the rest of the pumpkin family, with orange flesh inside the tough green skin. Peel using a potato peeler and add to stews or curries.

Pumpkin
These are usually more fibrous and watery than other squash. If sold in pieces, use within a few days as the flesh is more perishable once cut.

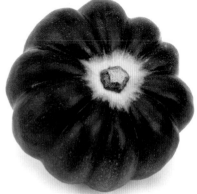

Butternut squash
A common variety of winter squash with a smooth, dense flesh, which is sweet and nutty. It will keep for a few weeks in a cool place. Good with lentils or coconut milk-based dishes.

Acorn squash
A mild-flavoured squash, slightly sweet, with firm, yellow-orange flesh. To prepare, cut in half, scoop out the seeds, then cut into quarters. Peel and cut to the size you require.

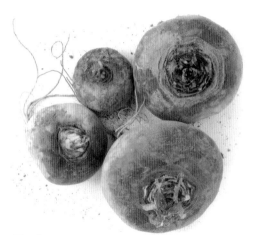

Carrot
Use either finely diced and sautéed with celery and onion to form a flavour base, or sliced to add colour and sweetness.

Turnip
The familiar top-shaped turnip is usually purple fading to white at the root. When small, the flavour is sweet and delicate.

Parsnip
The flavour of this creamy-beige root has hints of parsley and carrot, but with a slight sweetness and nuttiness. Use the scrubbed peel with other vegetable trimmings to make a winter vegetable stock.

Beetroot
The firm, juicy flesh of beetroot has an earthy, sweet flavour. It is best cooked with other red vegetables, or those that will absorb the seeping crimson juices.

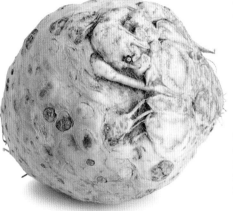

Celeriac
Celery root, or celeriac, has a thick, rough skin that conceals a crisp white flesh. It has a refreshing, slightly herbal flavour, combining the tastes of parsley and parsnip with celery.

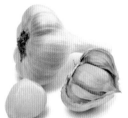

Shallot
They look like miniature onions, but shallots have a sweet, flowery flavour that does not overwhelm, and forms a rich flavour base for numerous sauces.

Garlic
Sauté garlic briefly at the beginning of a dish to add a layer of flavour; never cook until browned or it will taste bitter.

Sweet red onion
The juicy crimson and white flesh is noticeably sweet, although pungent when raw. Slow cooking caramelizes the juices and mellows the flavour.

Brown onion
The workhorse of the kitchen, the pungent brown onion is used in numerous savoury dishes, raw, fried, braised, stewed, boiled, or roasted.

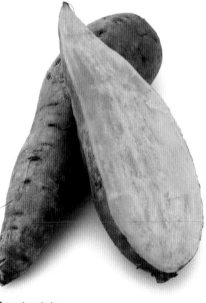

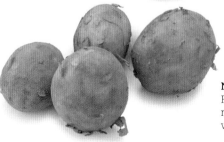

Potato
Choose waxy potatoes if you want them to hold their shape, or floury ones if you want them to dissolve and thicken the sauce.

Sweet potato
These have softer flesh than potatoes so will cook far quicker; add them to slow cooked dishes as a late addition. The taste is sweet, rather like squash.

New potato
Firm, with waxy flesh, these often don't need peeling and can be added to a dish whole. Use in summer casseroles.

Savoy cabbage
The attractively crinkled leaves are more loosely wrapped round the head than those of other cabbages and are more full-bodied in flavour.

Celery
A kitchen staple, celery makes a great base for casseroles and stews, along with carrot and onion. Trim the base and pull away any stringy bits.

Red cabbage
Offering beautiful, vibrant colour, red cabbage is sweeter than white, but the leaves are tougher, so they take longer to cook.

Curly kale
Exceptionally nutritious, the leaves have a rich, meaty flavour and robust texture. Kale will hold together quite well when slow cooked, or it can be added at the end.

Fennel
With its sweet, warm aniseed flavour and crisp texture, fennel makes a great vegetable for slow cooking. Either chop finely and sauté first with onion, or roughly chop and add to the pot. The flavour is subtler when cooked.

Poultry

The term "poultry" covers domesticated birds, including chicken, turkey, goose, guineafowl and duck (farmed duck is classified as game). This most versatile of meats works with most flavours and cooking methods. Whole birds or portions with the bone left in are ideal for slow cooking.

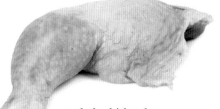

Whole chicken leg
Comprises the thigh and drumstick. A leg joint is good for slow cooking as the meat remains tender and juicy. Perfect for classics such as Coq au vin.

Chicken thigh
Sold skin on or off, bone-in, or boneless. Best with bone in for slow cooking as it keeps the meat tender and the taste is superior. When deboned, they are excellent stuffed and rolled up. Thighs are better than breast for slow cooking.

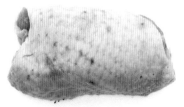

Whole chicken
These are perfect for poaching in flavoured liquid. The flesh becomes tender, moist, and silky and falls off the bone effortlessly. The bones can then be used for stock. Choose free range chicken, if you can, for ethical reasons and taste.

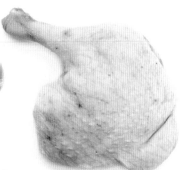

Duck leg
These have a superb flavour and rich dark meat. They take longer to cook than breast meat and have a little more sinew, but this makes them an incredibly tasty choice for slow cooking. Prick or slash the layer of skin and fat before browning in a pan.

Whole duck
It is better to joint these for slow cooking as they can be fatty. Ducks have a rich, dense meat that is best teamed with citrus fruits or spices that will cut through the fattiness of the meat.

Pork

Almost all pork cuts are suitable for slow cooking, but the cheaper, fattier varieties are the best as they provide the tastiest sauce. They go well with acidic-flavoured fruits, woody herbs, earthy vegetables, and lentils.

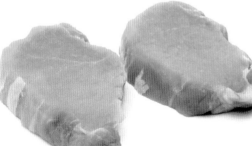

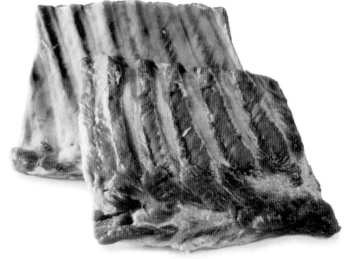

Pork leg
These are very lean so need careful cooking to prevent them from drying out. To cook as an escalope, leg steaks are beaten out very thinly.

Spare ribs
Trimmed ribs are sold as a rack or individually cut. Indivual ribs are easier to fit into a pot.

Rolled leg joint
Cuts from the lower leg, where the muscles are tougher, are suited to slow cooking. Pork leg meat can be bought cut into bite-sized pieces.

Belly slices
This is a fatty cut from the underside of the belly. Buy in whole pieces or slices. Slow cooking transforms it into tender meat. Goes well with Asian spices, hearty vegetables, or pulses.

Hock
The hock is the joint near the foot and is sometimes called pork knuckle. It is a cheap cut with lots of flavour that requires long and slow cooking.

Beef

There are many beef cuts suited to long slow cooking. These come from the forequarters and are less expensive than the leaner cuts. Choose beef that is a good, dark red colour, which has preferably been hung for 21 days. Beef responds well to marinating, as it adds depth of flavour to the finished dish and will tenderize the meat.

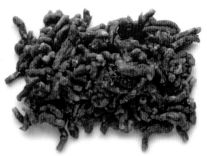

Minced beef
Forequarter (second grade) mince can be quite fatty but has good flavour. Minced shin needs the longest cooking. Steak mince from the back or leg is the leanest and most tender.

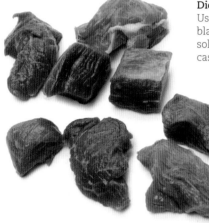

Diced braising steak
Usually lean chuck, blade, or flank. Often sold minced. Braise, casserole, or stew.

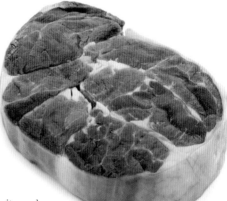

Shin of beef
Cut from the foreleg, it needs careful trimming. Dice and use for stews and casseroles.

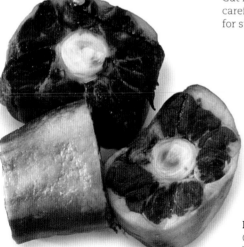

Oxtail
The tail is sold in chunks. The bones enrich sauces with their marrow. Stew, braise, or use in soup.

Brisket
Cut from the underside behind the front leg. Brisket needs long slow cooking because it has a lot of connective tissue, but has great flavour.

Lamb

As with all the best meats for slow cooking, the well-exercised parts of the animal make the choicest cuts. The high fat content in lamb meat makes it ideal for the slow cooker or casserole; slow cooking renders the meat meltingly tender and adds lots of flavour. Team lamb with sweet vegetables such as peas or fresh herbs such as mint, as these flavours cut through the fatty richness.

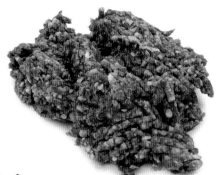

Minced lamb
This can be quite fatty and will add flavour and succulence to a dish. However, too much fat can make it greasy. Leg or shin will yield the leanest mince.

Neck fillet
Derived from the tender eye of the neck muscles, this cut of lamb is versatile and responds well to both high-heat quick cooking and long slow cooking. Cut into bite-sized pieces, or stuff it and cook it whole.

Shank
Slow, moist cooking is required to turn the sinews in the shank into a succulent jelly. Allow one shank per person. Foreleg shanks are slimmer than those from the back leg.

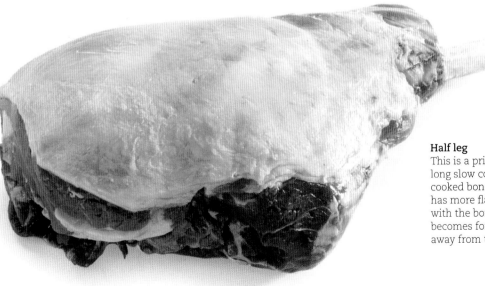

Half leg
This is a prime cut, but requires long slow cooking. It can be cooked bone in or bone out. It has more flavour when cooked with the bone in, as the meat becomes fork tender and falls away from the bone.

Fish

As a rule, fish is added towards the end of slow cooking as its delicate flesh needs only minimal time to cook. It adds a distinctive flavour to a slowly simmered sauce. Always choose sustainable fish.

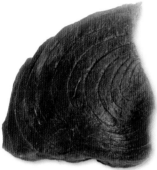

Tuna
Rich and full of flavour, tuna is robust enough to add to a slow cooked dish. Choose steaks that are fairly thick and try searing them first for extra flavour.

Halibut
Noted for its dense, firm, and low-fat white fillets, which have a mild taste. It is best served grilled or pan-fried with a flavoured butter.

Salmon
The flesh is firm, moist, and oily with a rich flavour. Choose chunky pieces and cut to a uniform size to add to the pot. Delicious added to a fish soup or stew.

Monkfish
With its dense texture, this is quite a "meaty" fish. It is a good choice for slow cooking as it won't fall apart easily. Monkfish has mildly flavoured, slightly chewy, white flesh.

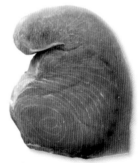

Swordfish
These meaty steaks have a similar texture to tuna and are ideal for using as a late addition to the pot.

Cod
This fish has white, chunky flakes with a delicate flavour. It needs very little cooking before the flesh is ready and turns opaque. If overcooked, cod will disintegrate and become chewy.

Haddock
This has a delicate, creamy, sweet flavour, similar to cod, and can be used instead of cod in recipes. Its delicate flesh needs only minimal cooking; add to the pot for a short time once the sauce is cooked.

Seafood

As with fish, seafood needs to be added late as it requires very little cooking. Seafood adds much flavour, texture, and protein to a dish and can transform an everyday sauce into a memorable meal.

Octopus
Slow cooking turns the meat tender and moist; undercooked, it can be chewy. You can buy it prepared or frozen, but be sure to defrost it thoroughly before adding to the pot. It is particularly good with a tomato-based sauce.

Squid
This requires either "fast flash" cooking or slow cooking in a simmering sauce to become tender. Like octopus, it is good in a tomato sauce. It has a mellow flavour so can take punchy sauces.

Clams
These have a delicate, sweet flavour with a texture similar to mussels. They need very little cooking and will steam open in minutes when added to a simmering sauce. A hearty, full-flavoured sauce makes a good accompaniment. Discard any clams that don't open after cooking.

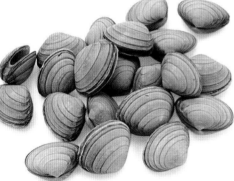

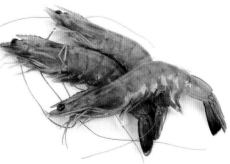

Prawns
Add prawns at the end of cooking as they will become tough and chewy if overcooked. The cooking time is dependent on their size. The shells make a tasty stock.

Mussels
They taste slightly salty, with an intense flavour of the sea. Add them to a dish late to prevent overcooking, which results in a rubbery texture. Once all the shells are open they are ready to eat.

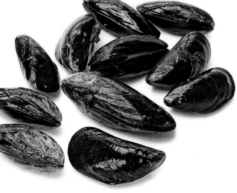

Most produce is suited to slow cooking, although some needs longer cooking than others. Knowing how to prepare fruits and vegetables correctly saves time and is key to a successful dish.

Preparing produce

Peeling and chopping garlic

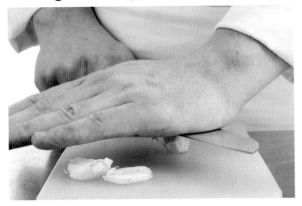 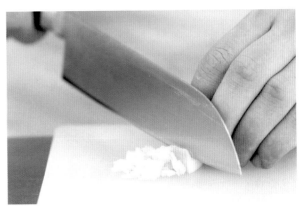

1 Place each garlic clove flat on a cutting board. Place the flat of a large knife blade on top and pound it with the heel of your hand.

2 Discard the skin and cut off the ends of each clove. Slice the clove into slivers lengthways, then cut across into tiny chunks. Collect the pieces into a pile and chop again for finer pieces.

Peeling and dicing onions

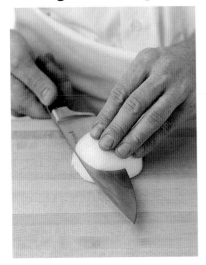 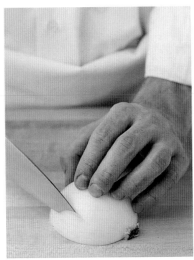 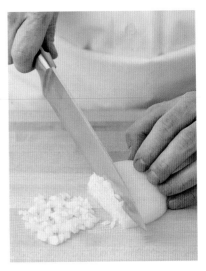

1 Cut the onion in half and peel it, leaving the root to hold the layers together. Make a few slices into the onion, but not through the root.

2 With the tip of your knife, slice down through the layers of onion vertically, cutting as close to the root as possible.

3 Cut across the vertical slices to produce an even dice. Use the root to hold the onion steady, then discard it when all the onion is diced.

Skinning and deseeding tomatoes

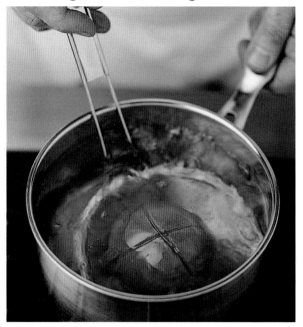

1 Remove the green stem, score an "X" in the skin of each tomato at the base, then immerse it in a pan of boiling water for 20 seconds, or until the skin loosens.

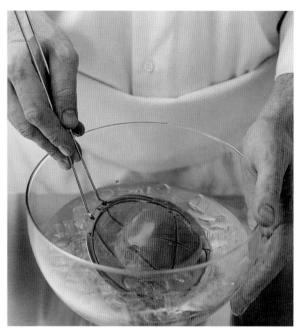

2 Using a slotted spoon, remove the tomato from the pan of boiling water and place it into a bowl of iced water to cool.

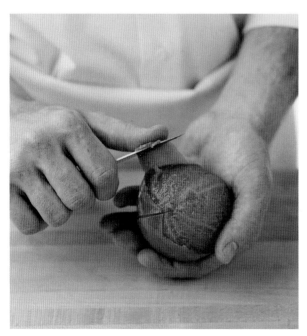

3 When cool enough to handle, use a paring knife to peel away the loosened skin.

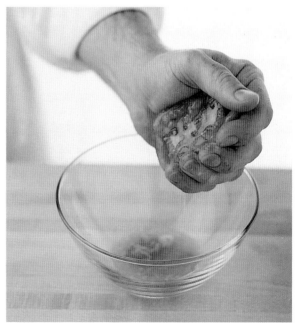

4 Cut each tomato in half and gently squeeze out the seeds over a bowl. Discard the seeds.

Roasting and peeling peppers

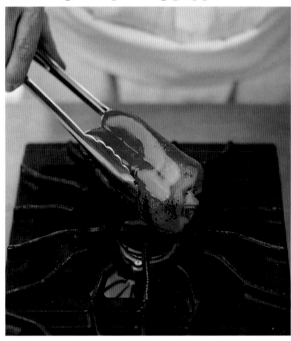

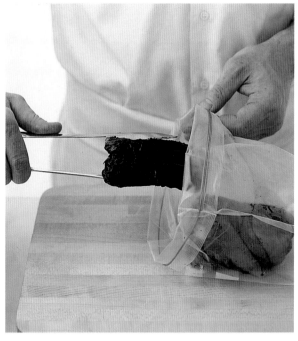

1 Using tongs, hold each pepper over an open flame to char the skin. Rotate the pepper to char it evenly.

2 Put the peppers into a plastic bag and seal tightly. Set the bag aside and allow the skins to loosen.

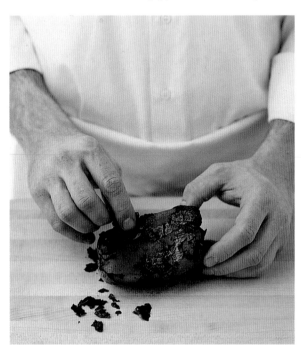

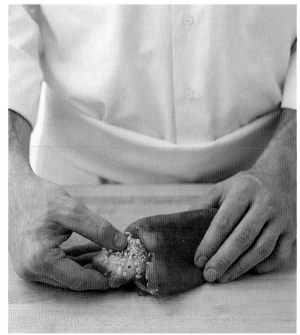

3 When the peppers have cooled completely, use your fingers to peel away the charred skin.

4 Pull off the stalk, keeping the core attached. Discard seeds and slice the flesh into strips, or roughly chop.

Coring and shredding cabbage

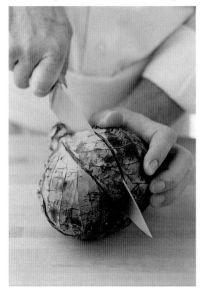

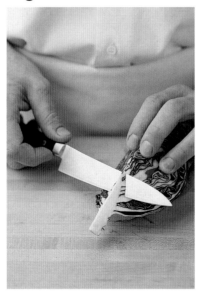

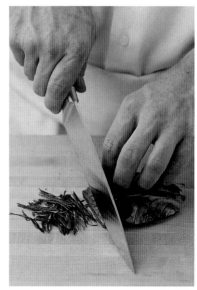

1 Hold the head of cabbage firmly on the cutting board and use a sharp knife to cut it in half, straight through the stalk end.

2 Cut the halves again through the stalk lengthways and slice out the core from each quarter.

3 Working with each quarter at a time, place the wedge cut-side down. Cut across the cabbage to shred it finely.

Trimming greens

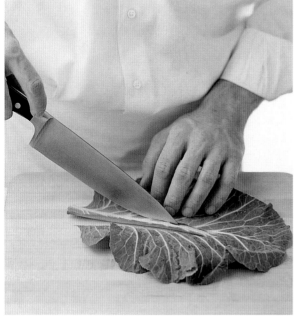

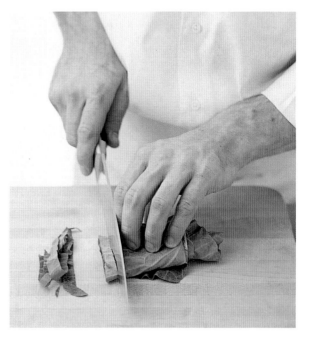

1 Discard all limp and discoloured leaves. Slice each leaf along both sides of the centre rib, then remove it and discard.

2 Working with a few leaves at a time, roll them loosely into a bunch. Cut across the roll to the desired width, making strips.

Peeling squashes

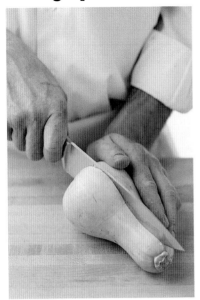 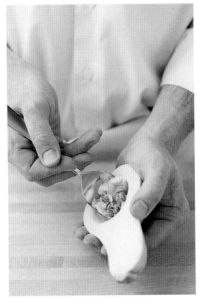 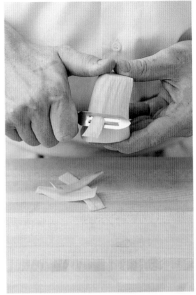

1 Holding the squash firmly, use a chef's knife to cut it lengthways in half, working from the stalk to the core.

2 Using a spoon, remove the seeds and fibres from each squash half and discard them.

3 Use a vegetable peeler or knife to remove the skin. Cut into pieces, then into chunks, or slice as required.

Rehydrating mushrooms

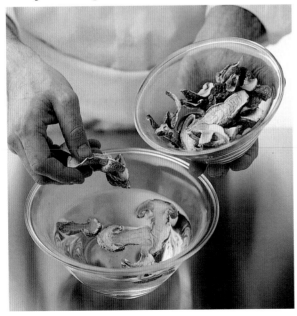 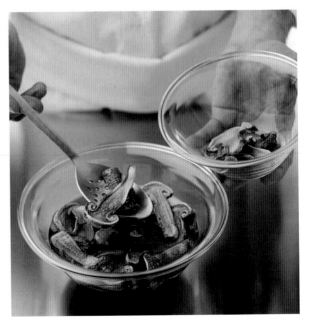

1 To rehydrate dried mushrooms, place the mushrooms – either wild or cultivated – into a bowl of hot water. Allow them to soak for at least 15 minutes.

2 Remove the mushrooms from the soaking liquid using a slotted spoon. If you plan to use the soaking liquid in your recipe, strain the liquid through a fine sieve, coffee filter, or muslin to remove any sand or grit.

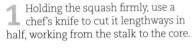

Herbs and spices are essential for adding aroma and flavour to a slow-cooked dish. Experience will teach you which spices to use with which foods, so use them sparingly at first. Add woody herbs, such as thyme and bay, at the beginning of slow cooking, but delicate ones, such as parsley and mint, are best added at the end as they can lose their potency. Chillies, on the other hand, can intensify on slow cooking.

Using herbs and spices

Making a bouquet garni

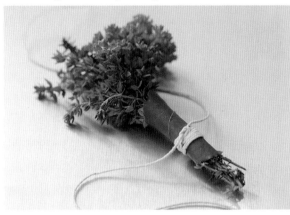

This is a bundle of herbs used to flavour a sauce. For a classic combination, tie sprigs of thyme and parsley and a bay leaf together. You could also include sage or rosemary.

Deseeding and cutting chillies

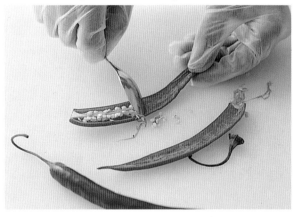

Slice chillies in half lengthways, then scrape out the seeds (this will reduce their heat, so leave if you wish). Slice or chop finely; wearing plastic gloves is a good idea.

Dry-roasting spices

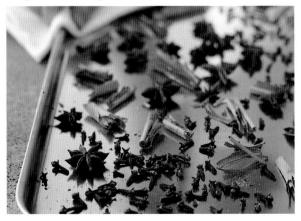

To dry-roast spices such as cloves, cinnamon, and star anise, place them in an oven preheated to 160°C (325°F/Gas 3), or fry them in a dry pan until lightly browned.

Frying spices in oil

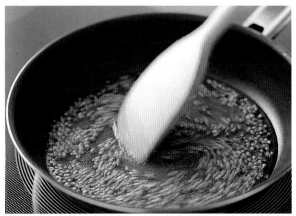

When spices are fried until lightly coloured, their flavour gets trapped in the oil. This is called tempering. The oil is used along with the spices at the start or end of cooking.

Versatile poultry works well with all types of slow cooking. The following techniques show you how to truss a bird for pot roasting, debone it, and portion it for stews and casseroles.

Preparing poultry

Trussing

This technique can appear quite fiddly but, once mastered, it only takes minutes to do. Trussing a bird before cooking allows it to hold its shape perfectly. It also helps cook it evenly, without overcooking any of the bony parts first. A poussin is shown here, but this works on other birds, too.

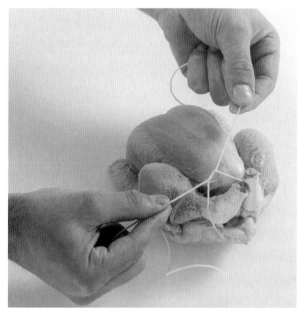

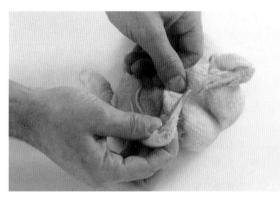

1 Season the insides of the bird with salt and pepper. Holding the bird breast-side down on a clean work surface, tuck the neck skin under the bird, and fold the wings over it.

2 Turn the bird over and pass a length of string under the tail end of the bird; tie a secure knot over the leg joints. Bring the strings along the sides of the body, between the breast and the legs, and loop them around the legs.

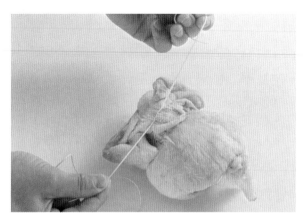

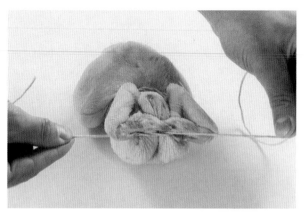

3 Turn the bird over so it is breast-side down again and tie the strings tightly under the body. Bring both ends of the string down between the sides of the body and the insides of the wings.

4 Tie the wing bones at the neck opening so they are tucked securely under the body. After cooking, cut the string to remove it.

Deboning poultry

If you prefer boneless meat, leg pieces (shown here) are better for slow cooking than the leaner breast meat. You may also wish to remove the bone to stuff the meat. Use a good, sharp knife and a series of shallow cuts to free the bone while preserving all the flesh. You can save the bones for stock.

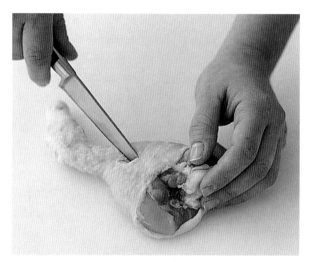

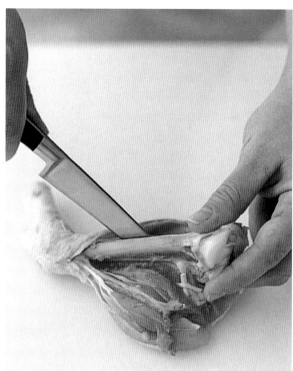

1 To debone a drumstick, start in the middle and insert the tip of your knife until you locate the bone. Slice along the bone in both directions to expose it fully.

2 Open the flesh and cut neatly around the bone using short strokes to free it completely from the flesh. Discard the bone, or use it to flavour stock.

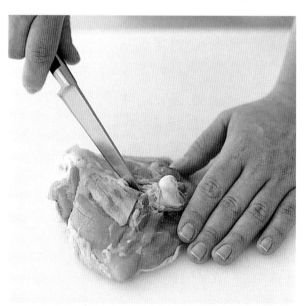

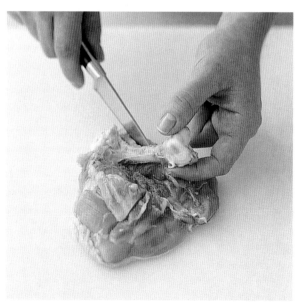

1 To debone a thigh, place the thigh skin-side down on a cutting board. Using a small, sharp knife, cut away the flesh to expose the thigh bone.

2 Cut an incision through the flesh, following the contour of the exposed bone. Cut around the bone to free it from the flesh. Discard the bone or use it for stock.

Jointing a chicken

This is a good skill to learn as it is often more economical to buy a whole chicken and joint it yourself than to buy expensive chicken pieces. The leftover bones and carcass can be used to make stock or soup. This jointing technique can be used for all poultry.

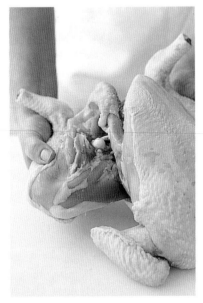

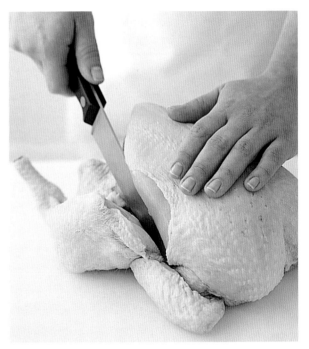

1 First, remove the wishbone. Using a sharp knife, scrape the flesh away from the wishbone, then use your fingers to twist and lift it free.

2 Place the bird breast-side up onto a cutting board. Cut down and through the thigh joint to separate the leg from the rest of the body.

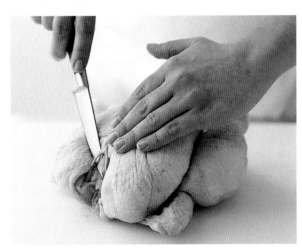

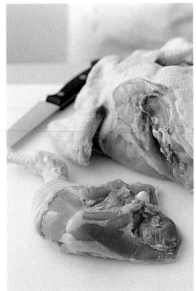

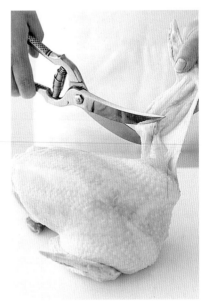

3 Bend the leg back to dislodge the leg joint. When the ball is free from the socket, you will hear a pop.

4 Cut any meat or skin still attached to the body. Repeat to remove the other leg. Each leg can be divided into a thigh and a drumstick.

5 Fully extend one wing, then use sharp poultry shears to cut off the winglet at the middle joint. Repeat to remove the other winglet.

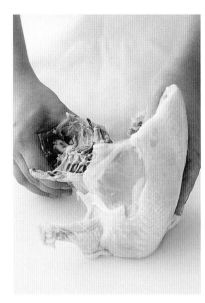

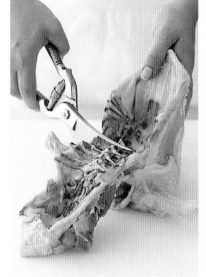

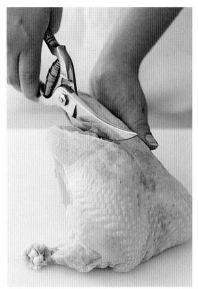

6 Grasp the backbone with your hands and break it from the crown (the 2 breasts and wings on the bone).

7 Using poultry shears, cut the lower end of the backbone from the remaining body.

8 Starting at the neck, cut all the way through the backbone to separate the breasts. The bird is now in 4 pieces.

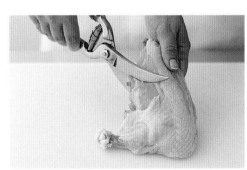

9 Use the poultry shears to cut each breast in half diagonally, producing one breast and one wing. Repeat to separate the other breast.

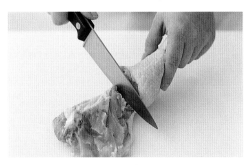

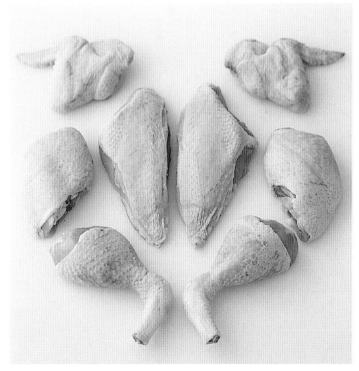

10 Cut each leg through the knee joint, above the drumstick that connects to the thigh, to separate. Now, there is one drumstick and one thigh. Repeat to separate the other leg.

11 The chicken is now cut into 8 pieces. Leg and thigh pieces are the choicest cuts for slow cooking, although breast pieces can work well for stewing when left on the bone. The wings contain juicy meat that is excellent for pot roasting.

Many cooks lack confidence when it comes to preparing fish, but all you need is the correct kit and a little know-how. An essential tool is a filleting knife, which is slightly flexible with a long blade. This makes it easy to remove the skin from fish and cut through the bones. Always buy good quality fresh fish and buy seafood on the day you will cook it. Clean seafood carefully so that nothing unwanted goes into the pot.

Preparing fish and seafood

Scaling and trimming fish

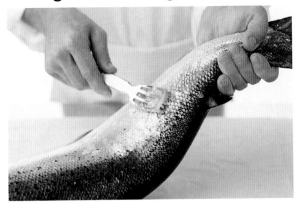

1 Lay the fish on top of a clean work surface. Holding the fish by the tail, scrape the scales off with a fish scaler or the blade of a chef's knife, using strokes towards the head.

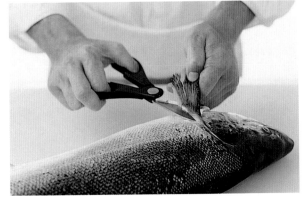

2 Once the fish is descaled, use kitchen scissors to remove the dorsal (back) fin, the belly fins, and the two fins on either side of the head.

Filleting and skinning a fish

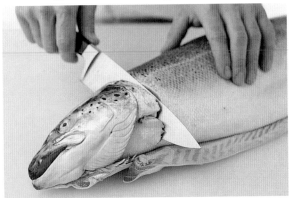

1 Don't scale a fish if you plan to skin it. To fillet, gut the fish through the stomach, then cut into the head at an angle, just behind the gills, until you reach the backbone. Move to the top side of the backbone and, starting near the gills, cut down the length of one side of the backbone.

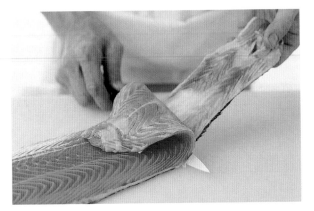

2 Turn over, and repeat the cut on the other side of the backbone. Place the fillet skin-side down onto a clean work surface. Insert a filleting knife into the flesh of the fish near the tail end. Turn the blade at an angle almost parallel to the skin and cut off the flesh, while holding the skin taut.

Preparing mussels

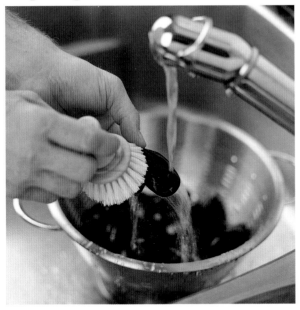

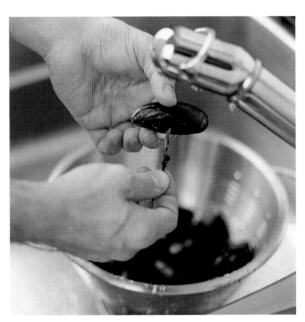

1 Discard any mussels that are broken or wide open. In the sink, scrub the mussels under cold, running water. Rinse away grit or sand and remove any barnacles with a small, sharp knife.

2 To remove the "beard", pinch the dark, stringy piece between your fingers, pull it away from the mussel, and discard. If a mussel is not tightly closed, tap it to check it is fresh; if it doesn't close when you tap it, discard it.

Peeling and deveining prawns

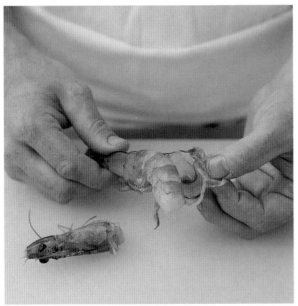

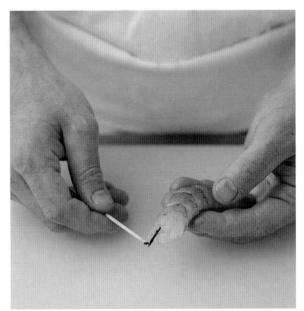

1 Remove the head and legs by pulling them off with your fingers, then peel away the shells. Save the shells for stock, if you like.

2 Using the tip of a paring knife or cocktail stick, hook the vein where the head was and gently pull it away from the body.

Slow cooking provides a convenient one-pot cooking method, but with most dishes there are a few stages of cooking that are needed first, such as marinating, browning the meat, or sautéing vegetables. Each of these techniques adds depth of flavour to the finished dish. Deglazing during cooking is vital for enhancing the taste of your sauce, while reducing and thickening are great troubleshooting techniques for thin sauces.

Essential recipe techniques

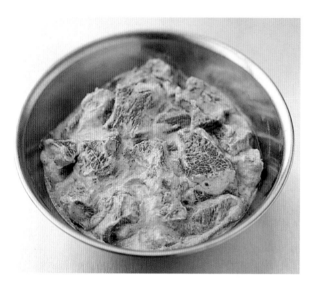

Marinating

A marinade is a mixture that meat or fish is steeped in before cooking, and should be made up of acidic ingredients such as wine, citrus juice or vinegar, and salt. Soaking the meat is called marinating, a process that tenderizes and enhances flavour in tougher, cheaper cuts. Trim the meat before marinating and cut it to the required size. Natural yogurt can also be used as a marinade and is a common tenderizer for chicken, turkey, or seafood, although it can be used for red meat as well. Spices, herbs, and aromatic vegetables such as garlic, onion, and ginger are often included in marinades to add extra flavour. Make sure the meat is immersed in the marinade, then leave it in the refrigerator to marinate for 4–12 hours.

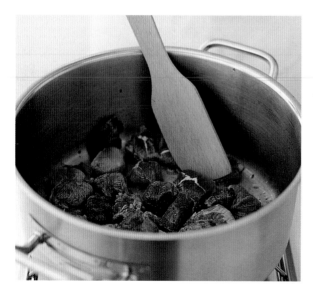

Browning

This technique caramelizes the natural sugars that are in meat and turns it a rich golden colour. Browning adds flavour and depth to your dish, so it is well worth doing at the beginning of the recipe before adding the meat to the other ingredients. Season the meat and add it to a little hot oil or butter in a pan and cook at a medium-high heat. Leave the meat to cook undisturbed for a few minutes. You will know it is ready when it comes away from the bottom of the pan easily. When the underside is golden, turn and cook the other side. Remove the meat and set it aside while you prepare the rest of the ingredients. You could dust the meat in seasoned flour before browning, as it is a good way to help thicken the consistency of the sauce.

Sautéing

This requires high heat and a good heavy-based pan. Sautéing vegetables enables their natural water content to evaporate, thus concentrating their flavour. Heat some oil or butter, add the vegetables to the pan, and cook until they start to caramelize and soften. This takes no longer than around 5–8 minutes, depending on the vegetables you are cooking. Move them around the pan to prevent burning. Always cook the hardest vegetables first as these will take longer. Don't overcrowd the pan or the vegetables will sweat rather than sauté.

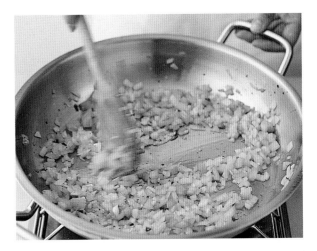

Deglazing

The sauce is all-important as it can make or break the finished dish. Pan sauces and gravies are made from deglazed caramelized juices released from roasted or fried meat, poultry, and vegetables. In slow cooking, this technique is used often after browning and sautéing. Remove the food from the pan and spoon off excess fat, then deglaze the caramelized juices by adding stock, water, or wine. Stir to loosen the particles and incorporate them into the liquid. Reduce and finish as required. Making a sauce like this gives a richness and depth of flavour that cannot be achieved just by simmering ingredients.

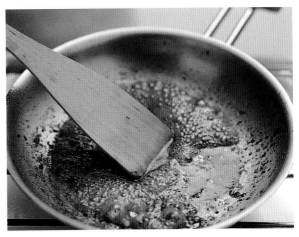

Reducing and thickening

When a sauce is too thin, it can be either reduced or thickened to improve its flavour and texture. Reducing decreases the sauce's volume through evaporation and intensifies its flavour. To reduce, cook in an uncovered pan over a high heat, stirring occasionally. Add stock and bring back to boil, then boil, uncovered, for about 20 minutes to reduce again by half, regularly skimming off any impurities. Thickening gives sauces extra body and consistency. There are different ways to do this. A simple method is to dissolve cornflour in water and add the mixture to the simmering dish. You could also add a roux – a mixture of flour and water – stirring it into the simmering sauce and cooking to prevent it from turning the sauce lumpy.

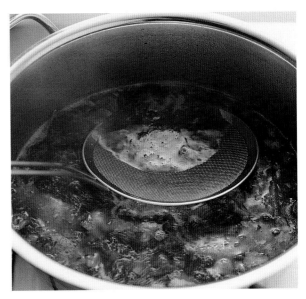

Using your slow cooker is a simple and efficient way to make stock – the liquid won't evaporate and boil dry, so you can leave it unattended. Save the carcass or bones from poultry, meat, or fish when preparing a dish, then add them to the slow cooker with water and flavourings and leave it to simmer overnight. Stock freezes well, so if you are not using it straight away, let it cool and freeze it for up to 1 month.

Making stock in the slow cooker

Vegetable stock

1 Save scraps, peelings, stalks, tops, and ends from vegetables such as onion, carrot, celery, leek, and fennel to use as the base of your stock.

2 Add the vegetable scraps to the slow cooker. You can also add any herbs you may have, such as parsley stalks and a bay leaf, along with a few black peppercorns and a pinch of salt.

3 Boil enough water to cover all the ingredients, then pour this into the slow cooker. Cover with the lid, and cook on auto/low for 6–8 hours. Skim the stock halfway through the cooking time, if needed. Strain the stock and allow to cool before storing in the refrigerator or freezer.

Meat stock

1 Add a chicken carcass or beef bones to the slow cooker with a handful of raw vegetables such as carrot tops, celery, and onion.

2 Add some black peppercorns and a pinch of salt to the slow cooker, along with herbs such as parsley or a bay leaf, if you wish.

3 Boil enough water to cover all the ingredients, then pour this into the slow cooker. Cover with the lid, and cook on auto/low for 6–8 hours. Skim the stock halfway through the cooking time, if needed. Strain the stock and allow to cool before storing in the refrigerator or freezer.

Fish stock

1 Ask your fishmonger for some fish heads, or use leftovers from another dish. Choose white fish such as sea bass or haddock, but avoid oily fish as their stonger flavour will taint the stock.

2 Add the fish scraps to the slow cooker along with some fresh herbs, such as thyme, and some fennel scraps or onion.

3 Pour over enough boiling water to cover all the ingredients, cover with the lid, and cook on auto/low for 6–8 hours. Skim the stock halfway through the cooking time, if needed. Strain the stock and allow to cool before storing in the refrigerator or freezer.

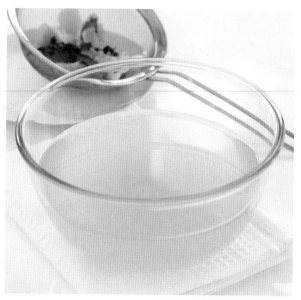

Fish stock

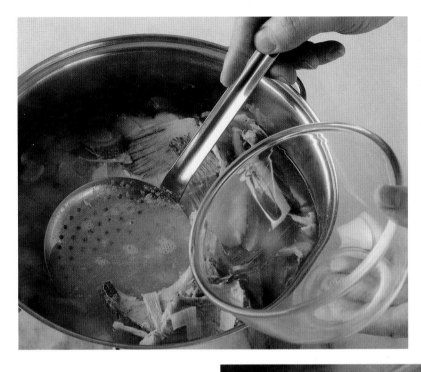

Skimming stock

When making stock, quite often a layer of frothy "scum" will appear on the surface. To skim it off, use a ladle or a metal spoon to scoop it away and then discard it. You may find you need to do this a few times during cooking. Meat and fish stocks are most likely to need skimming.

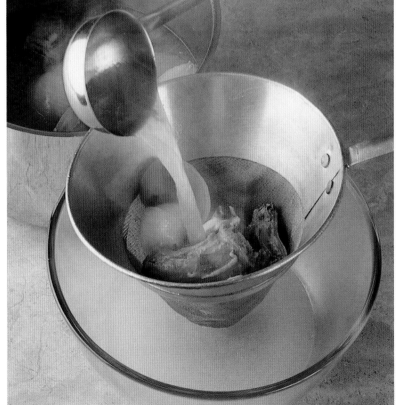

Straining stock

Once the stock has finished cooking, strain it straight away; don't leave it sitting. To strain the stock, turn the slow cooker off then lift out the inner pot. Carefully strain the stock liquid into a jug or bowl through a fine nylon mesh sieve, or you could line a sieve with muslin. It is easiest to do this a ladleful at a time. Discard any bones, carcass, and vegetables used and leave the stock to cool.

Adding dumplings, a cobbler topping, or breadcrumbs to a stew or casserole can make a dish inviting, more filling, and substantial. All are easy to prepare while your dish is simmering; simply add them to the pot to get a complete one-pot meal without any additional cooking.

Extras and toppings

Suet dumplings

1 The secret to light and fluffy dumplings lies in handling the dough as little as possible. Add 150g (5½oz) shredded suet (either regular or vegetarian) and 150g (5½oz) self-raising flour to a bowl and mix together with your hands. Season well with salt and pepper.

2 If you wish, some extra flavourings could be added to the mixture at this point, such as 30g (1oz) freshly grated Parmesan cheese, 1 tsp mustard or horseradish, or 1–2 tsp fresh chopped herbs such as parsley, thyme, and rosemary. Mix any flavourings into the dry ingredients.

3 Make a well in the middle of the flour mixture and slowly drizzle in cold water a little at a time. Mix with your hands until the mixture starts to come together and leaves the sides of the bowl easily.

4 Turn out onto a lightly floured board and roll into a sausage shape. Form into 6 large or 12 small dumplings (they will double in size as they cook). For the slow cooker, add the dumplings in for the last 45–60 minutes of cooking. For the traditional method, add them to the casserole for the last 30 minutes of cooking. They should be just immersed in the liquid and covered with a lid.

Non-suet dumplings

1 This recipe uses butter instead of suet to make a light, moist version of the dumpling. Add 100g (3½oz) white breadcrumbs, 100g (3½oz) self-raising flour, and 140g (5oz) butter to a food processor and whiz into a crumb mixture. You could also add some extra flavourings to the food processor, if you like, such as freshly grated Parmesan cheese, mustard or horseradish, or fresh chopped herbs like parsley, thyme, and rosemary.

2 Add 2 eggs to the food processor and season with salt and pepper. Whiz again until the mixture comes together as a moist dough.

3 Turn the dough out onto a lightly floured board and roll into 6 large or 12 small balls (keep in mind that the dumplings will double in size as they cook). For the slow cooker, add the dumplings to the pot for the last 45–60 minutes of cooking. For the traditional method, add the dumplings to the casserole for the last 30 minutes of cooking. They should be just immersed in the liquid and covered with a lid.

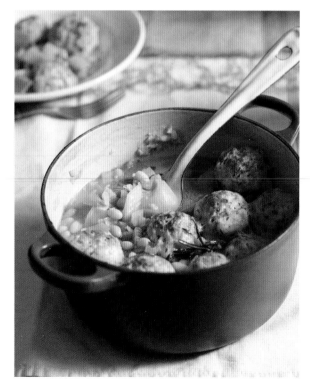

Vegetable casserole (p100) with herby suet dumplings

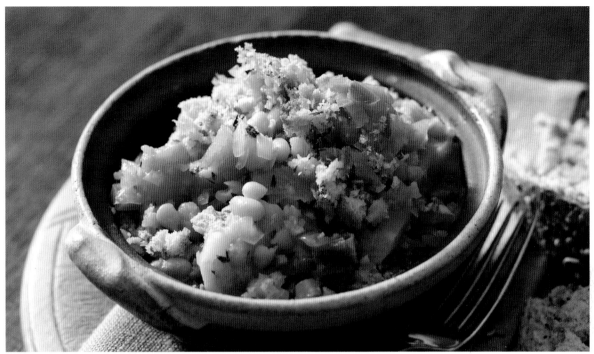

Pumpkin and parsnip cassoulet (p102) with breadcrumb topping.

Breadcrumbs

1 Using a food processor, whiz 2 slices of torn bread into coarse crumbs. Add any flavourings of your choice, such as herbs or grated cheese, and whiz again. If your recipe calls for fresh breadcrumbs, then they can be used at this stage. For the slow cooker, lightly toast the breadcrumbs in a dry frying pan; sprinkle over, or carefully fold into, the finished dish. For the traditional method, sprinkle into the casserole and cook in the oven for the last 30 minutes of cooking; remove the lid for the last 10 minutes, or until the topping is golden.

2 For fine, golden breadcrumbs, spread them onto a baking tray and put in the oven at 200°C (400°F/ Gas 6) for about 10 minutes until golden. Remove, tip back into the food processor, and whiz again until fine. You can add any flavourings at this time, if you wish, such as fresh herbs or grated cheese. Use to top the dish for the last hour of cooking for both the slow cooker and for the traditional method.

3 If you are not using the breadcrumbs immediately, they can be frozen for up to 3 months. They don't require defrosting before use.

Cobblers

1 A cobbler topping is a small savoury scone that makes a wholesome and filling dish. Use them to top chicken, beef, lamb, or vegetable stews and casseroles. Put 200g (7oz) sifted self-raising flour and salt and pepper in a bowl and mix together. Add any flavourings, such as grated cheese, chopped sun-dried tomatoes or olives, or ground walnuts to the dry ingredients, if you wish.

2 Cut 100g (3½oz) butter into cubes and rub it into the ingredients in the bowl with your fingertips until the mixture resembles breadcrumbs. Add 2 lightly beaten eggs and mix until the dough comes together, then add 4 tbsp milk a little at a time, mixing until it becomes a soft dough.

3 Turn the dough out onto a lightly floured board and roll out so it is fairly thick. Using a 2.5cm (1in) metal cutter, cut out 6 rounds. For the slow cooker, add the cobblers to the top of the dish for the last hour of cooking. For the traditional method, add the cobblers to the top of the casserole, brush the tops with the milk, and cook in the oven, uncovered, for the last 30–45 minutes of cooking.

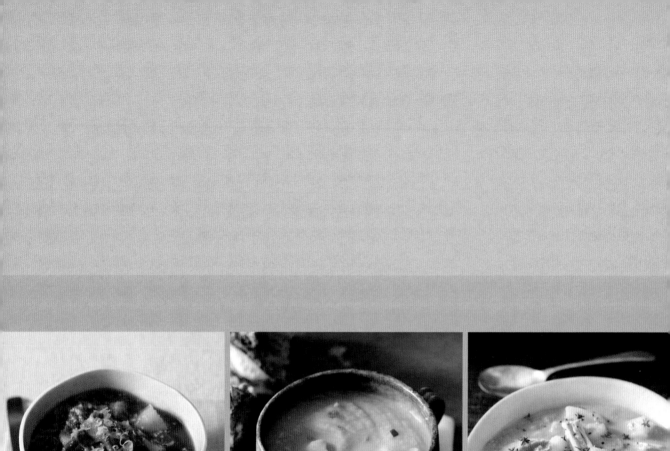

Soups & broths

This soup is just as good in summer made with fresh tomatoes and basil pesto stirred through it as it is in winter with added canned beans to bulk it out. It is excellent for freezing.

Provençal vegetable soup

◎ **SERVES** 4–6   ❄ **FREEZE** UP TO 3 MONTHS

1 tbsp olive oil
1 onion, finely chopped
salt and freshly ground black pepper
3 garlic cloves, finely chopped
2 celery sticks, finely chopped
2 carrots, peeled and roughly chopped
sprig of tarragon, leaves finely chopped
2 sprigs of rosemary

400g can tomatoes, blended until smooth
900ml (1½ pints) hot vegetable stock, for
  both methods
3 potatoes, peeled and chopped
  into bite-sized pieces
325g (11oz) green dwarf beans or French or fine green
  beans, trimmed and chopped into bite-sized pieces
30g (1oz) Parmesan cheese, grated (optional)

in the slow cooker   🕑 **PREP** 15 MINS   **COOK** 10 MINS PRECOOKING;
AUTO/LOW 8 HRS OR HIGH 4 HRS

1 Preheat the slow cooker, if required. Heat the oil in a large heavy-based pan over a medium heat, add the onion, and cook for 3–4 minutes until soft. Season with salt and pepper, then stir through the garlic and celery and cook for a further 5 minutes or until the celery is soft.

2 Stir in the carrots, tarragon, and rosemary and cook for a minute before transferring everything to the slow cooker. Stir in the puréed tomatoes and stock and cook on auto/low for 8 hours or on high for 4 hours. Add the potatoes for the last 15 minutes of cooking.

3 When the potatoes are soft, add the beans and cook for 10 minutes, or until they are cooked but retain a bite. Taste and season, remove the rosemary, and ladle into warmed large shallow bowls. Sprinkle over the Parmesan, if using, and serve with some crusty French bread.

traditional method   🕑 **PREP** 15 MINS   **COOK** 1 HR

1 Heat the oil in a large heavy-based pan over a medium heat, add the onion, and cook for 3–4 minutes until soft. Season with salt and pepper, then stir through the garlic and celery and cook for a further 5 minutes or until the celery is soft.

2 Stir in the carrots, tarragon, and rosemary and cook for a minute, then tip in the puréed tomatoes and a little stock, and bring to the boil. Add the remaining stock and return to the boil, then reduce to a simmer, partially cover with the lid, and cook gently for about 45 minutes. If more liquid is needed, top up with a little hot water. Add the potatoes for the last 15 minutes of cooking.

3 When the potatoes are soft, add the beans and cook for a further 10 minutes, or until they are cooked but retain a bite. Taste and season, remove the rosemary, and ladle into warmed large shallow bowls. Sprinkle over the Parmesan, if using, and serve with some crusty French bread.

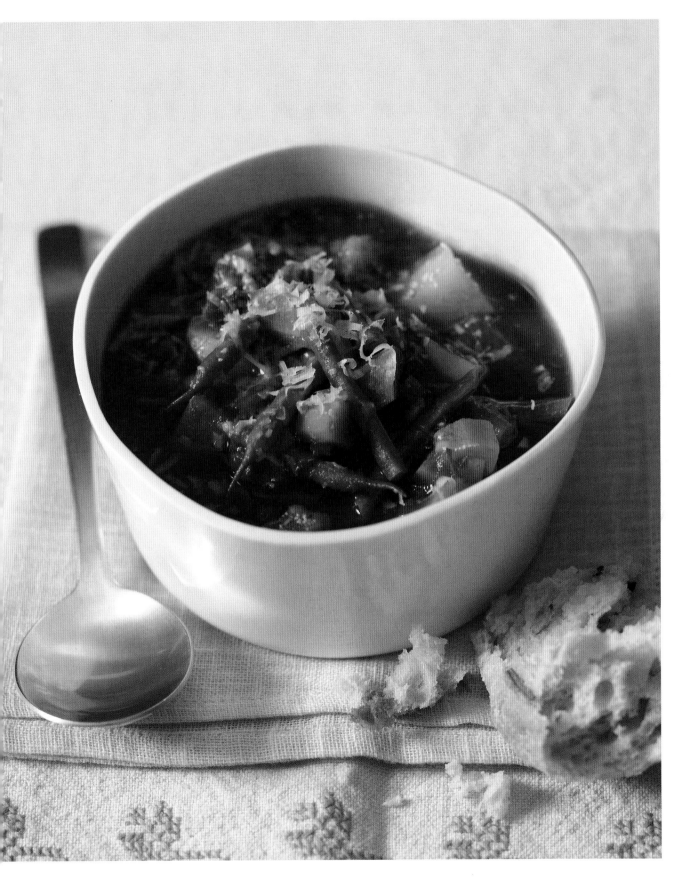

Lots of complex flavours make up this warming broth. The water chestnuts add an unexpected texture, and the chicken and prawns add plenty of protein, making it a substantial dish.

Asian chicken and prawn broth with ginger and coriander

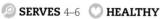 **SERVES** 4–6 **HEALTHY**

1.2 litres (2 pints) hot chicken stock, for both methods
salt and freshly ground black pepper
1 tbsp dark soy sauce
3 tbsp fish sauce (nam pla)
3 tbsp mirin
1 tsp tahini
2 garlic cloves, finely chopped
5cm (2in) piece of fresh root ginger, peeled and sliced into fine strips

½ tsp dried chilli flakes
225g can bamboo shoots, drained and rinsed
225g can water chestnuts, drained and rinsed
125g (4½oz) button mushrooms, whole or larger ones halved
2 skinless chicken breasts, finely sliced
bunch of spring onions, finely chopped
bunch of coriander leaves
250g pack of ready-cooked small prawns or shrimps

in the slow cooker **PREP** 15 MINS **COOK** HIGH 2–2½ HRS

1 Preheat the slow cooker, if required. Put everything into the slow cooker except the spring onions, coriander, and prawns and add 300ml (10fl oz) of hot water.

2 Cover with the lid and cook on high for 2–2½ hours, stirring through the spring onions, coriander, and prawns for the last 20 minutes of cooking. Taste and season as required, and ladle into warmed bowls while piping hot.

traditional method **PREP** 15 MINS **COOK** 1 HR

1 Put the stock into a large heavy-based pan, season with salt and pepper, and add a further 600ml (1 pint) of hot water. Add the soy sauce, fish sauce, mirin, and tahini and bring to the boil.

2 Reduce to a simmer and add the garlic, ginger, and chilli flakes together with the bamboo shoots, water chestnuts, and mushrooms. Stir, then add the chicken, cover with the lid, and cook gently for 40 minutes. Top up with hot water if necessary.

3 Taste and adjust seasoning as required, then stir through the spring onions and coriander leaves, and simmer on a low heat for a further 10 minutes. Finally, add the prawns and simmer for 5 minutes. Ladle into warmed bowls while piping hot.

The secret of a good French onion soup is to let the onions caramelize slowly so they become wonderfully sweet.
If you like, you could use a dry cider instead of the wine.

French onion soup

⊚ **SERVES** 4 ❄ **FREEZE** UP TO 1 MONTH, WITHOUT THE BREAD OR CHEESE

30g (1oz) butter
1 tbsp sunflower oil
675g (1½lb) onions, thinly sliced
1 tsp caster sugar
salt and freshly ground black pepper
120ml (4fl oz) dry white wine
2 tbsp plain flour

1 litre (1¾ pints) hot beef stock for the slow cooker
    (1.5 litres /2¾ pints for the traditional method)
4 tbsp brandy
1 garlic clove, chopped in half
4 slices of baguette, about 2cm (¾in) thick, toasted
115g (4oz) Gruyère or Emmental cheese, grated

in the slow cooker 🕐 **PREP** 20 MINS **COOK** 45 MINS PRECOOKING;
AUTO/LOW 4–6 HRS OR **HIGH** 2–3 HRS

1 Melt the butter with the oil in a large heavy-based pan over a low heat. Stir together the onions and sugar, and season with salt and pepper. Press a piece of wet greaseproof paper over the surface and cook, stirring occasionally, uncovered, for 40 minutes, or until the onions are rich and dark golden brown. Take care that they do not stick and burn at the bottom.

2 Preheat the slow cooker, if required. Remove the paper and stir in the wine. Increase the heat to medium and stir for 5 minutes, or until the onions are glazed. Sprinkle with the flour and stir for 2 minutes. Stir in the stock and bring to the boil. Transfer everything to the slow cooker, cover with the lid, and cook on auto/low for 4–6 hours or on high for 2–3 hours. Taste and adjust the seasoning, if necessary.

3 Preheat the grill on its highest setting. Divide the soup between 4 flameproof bowls and stir 1 tbsp of brandy into each. Rub the garlic clove over the toast and place 1 slice in each bowl. Sprinkle with the cheese and grill for 2–3 minutes, or until the cheese is bubbling and golden. Serve at once.

traditional method 🕐 **PREP** 10 MINS **COOK** 1½ HRS

1 Melt the butter with the oil in a large heavy-based pan over a low heat. Stir together the onions and sugar, and season with salt and pepper. Press a piece of wet greaseproof paper over the surface and cook, stirring occasionally, uncovered, for 40 minutes, or until the onions are rich and dark golden brown. Take care that they do not stick and burn at the bottom.

2 Remove the paper and stir in the wine. Increase the heat to medium and stir for 5 minutes, or until the onions are glazed. Sprinkle with the flour and stir for 2 minutes. Stir in the stock and bring to the boil. Reduce the heat to low, cover with the lid, and leave the soup to simmer for 30 minutes. Taste and adjust the seasoning, if necessary.

3 Meanwhile, preheat the grill on its highest setting. Divide the soup between 4 flameproof bowls and stir 1 tbsp of brandy into each. Rub the garlic clove over the toast and place 1 slice in each bowl. Sprinkle with the cheese and grill for 2–3 minutes, or until the cheese is bubbling and golden. Serve at once.

This is a substantial meal-in-one that is full of complex flavours.
It's also one of those dishes that tastes better when reheated,
so if you have the time, make it a day ahead and reheat to eat.

Moroccan harira soup

⊙ **SERVES** 4–6 ❋ **FREEZE** UP TO 1 MONTH

1 tbsp olive oil
1 red onion, finely chopped
salt and freshly ground black pepper
3 garlic cloves, finely chopped
1 celery stick, chopped
675g (1½lb) shoulder or shank of lamb, cut
  into bite-sized pieces
1 tsp ground turmeric
1 tsp ground cinnamon
5cm (2in) piece of fresh root ginger, peeled
  and finely chopped

900ml (1½ pints) hot vegetable stock
  for the slow cooker (1.4 litres/2½ pints for
  the traditional method)
125g (4½oz) green or brown lentils, rinsed
  well and picked over for any stones
400g can chickpeas, drained and rinsed
1 tsp harissa paste
few sprigs of coriander, leaves only, to serve

in the slow cooker 🕒 **PREP** 25 MINS **COOK** 25–30 MINS PRECOOKING; AUTO/LOW 8 HRS

1 Preheat the slow cooker, if required. Heat the oil in a large flameproof casserole over a medium heat, add the onion, and cook for 3–4 minutes until soft. Season with salt and pepper, then stir through the garlic and celery and cook for a further 6–10 minutes until the celery is soft.

2 Add the lamb, turmeric, cinnamon, and ginger. Increase the heat a little, stir until the lamb is coated, and cook for 6–10 minutes until the lamb is no longer pink. Add a ladleful of stock and bring to the boil. Stir through the lentils and chickpeas, turning them to coat evenly, add the remaining stock, and bring back to the boil.

3 Transfer everything to the slow cooker. Stir through the harissa paste, cover with the lid, and cook on auto/low for 8 hours. Ladle into warmed bowls, top with coriander leaves, and serve with lemon wedges on the side.

traditional method 🕒 **PREP** 25 MINS **COOK** 2 HRS

1 Heat the oil in a large flameproof casserole over a medium heat, add the onion, and cook for 3–4 minutes until soft. Season with salt and pepper, then stir through the garlic and celery and cook for a further 6–10 minutes until the celery is soft.

2 Add the lamb, turmeric, cinnamon, and ginger. Increase the heat a little, stir until the lamb is coated, and cook for 6–10 minutes until the lamb is no longer pink. Add a ladleful of stock and bring to the boil. Stir through the lentils and chickpeas, turning them to coat evenly, add the remaining stock, and bring back to the boil.

3 Reduce to a gentle simmer and cook for 1–1½ hours until the lamb is meltingly tender. Check occasionally that it's not drying out, topping up with a little hot water if needed. Stir through the harissa paste and cook for a few more minutes. Ladle into warmed bowls, top with coriander leaves, and serve with lemon wedges on the side.

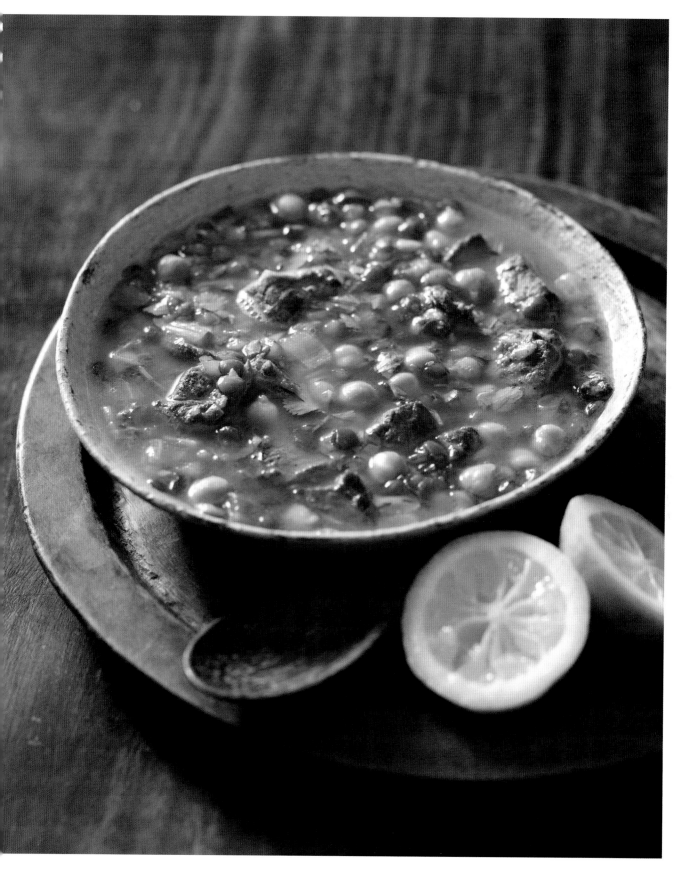

The broth in this recipe has a rich beef flavour, with the barley and dumplings adding plenty of texture and variety. They also turn the soup into a hearty, warming meal.

Beef broth with parmesan dumplings

⊙ **SERVES** 6　❄ **FREEZE** UP TO 3 MONTHS, WITHOUT THE DUMPLINGS　♡ **HEALTHY**

1.1kg (2½lb) brisket on the bone, cut into small
  pieces (ask your butcher to do this for you)
salt and freshly ground black pepper
75g (2½oz) pearl barley
1 onion, roughly chopped
3 celery sticks, finely chopped
3 garlic cloves, finely chopped
4 carrots, peeled and sliced
3 small turnips, peeled and diced
4 tomatoes

few sprigs of flat-leaf parsley, leaves only,
  finely chopped

FOR THE PARMESAN DUMPLINGS
60g (2oz) breadcrumbs
60g (2oz) Parmesan cheese, grated,
  plus extra, to serve
pinch of grated nutmeg
1 egg

in the slow cooker　⊙ **PREP** 15 MINS　**COOK** AUTO/LOW 6–8 HRS

1 Preheat the slow cooker, if required. Put the beef bones, with enough water to cover them (about 900ml/1½ pints), and all the other soup ingredients, into the slow cooker, including seasoning. Cover with the lid and cook on auto/low for 6–8 hours. Remove the beef bones and then remove the meat, chop if needed, and return it to the slow cooker.

2 Meanwhile, prepare the dumplings. Mix together the breadcrumbs, Parmesan cheese, and nutmeg, season well, and then mix in the egg. Turn the mixture out onto a floured board and knead for a couple of minutes, then form into tiny balls. Add them to the slow cooker for the last 10 minutes of cooking. Ladle the soup into warmed shallow bowls and sprinkle with Parmesan cheese and parsley. Serve with crusty bread rolls.

traditional method　⊙ **PREP** 15 MINS　**COOK** 2½ HRS

1 Put the beef bones into a large heavy-based pan and cover with 1.4 litres (2½ pints) of water. Season well with salt and pepper, and bring to the boil. Skim off any scum that builds up, reduce the heat, cover with the lid, and let the broth simmer gently for about 1½ hours. Add the pearl barley, onion, celery, garlic, carrots, turnips, and tomatoes, partially cover with the lid, and cook for a further 45 minutes, or until the pearl barley is tender. Top up with a little hot water, if needed.

2 Meanwhile, prepare the dumplings. Mix together the breadcrumbs, Parmesan cheese, and nutmeg, season well, and then mix in the egg. Turn the mixture out onto a floured board and knead for a couple of minutes, then form into tiny balls.

3 When the meat is cooked, use a slotted spoon to take the beef bones out of the pan. Remove the meat, chop if needed, and return it to the pan. Add the dumplings to the soup and cook gently for about 5 minutes, then ladle it into warmed shallow bowls and sprinkle with Parmesan cheese and parsley. Serve with crusty bread rolls.

This soup will make a really substantial meal on its own. Make it without the chorizo if you are feeding vegetarians, but add a little smoked paprika to replace the smoky flavour.

Cajun mixed bean soup

SERVES 4–6   **FREEZE** UP TO 3 MONTHS

1 tbsp olive oil
1 onion, finely chopped
salt and freshly ground black pepper
3 garlic cloves, finely chopped
2 celery sticks, finely chopped
200g (7oz) chorizo, cubed
pinch of dried chilli flakes

few sprigs of thyme
2 sweet potatoes, peeled and cubed
2 yellow peppers, deseeded and roughly chopped
2 x 400g cans adzuki beans, drained and rinsed
400g can kidney beans, drained and rinsed
450ml (15fl oz) hot vegetable stock for the slow cooker (900ml/1½ pints for the traditional method)

in the slow cooker   PREP 10 MINS   COOK 25 MINS PRECOOKING; AUTO/LOW 8 HRS OR HIGH 3 HRS

1 Preheat the slow cooker, if required. Heat the oil in a large heavy-based pan over a medium heat, add the onion, and cook for 3–4 minutes until soft. Season with salt and pepper, stir through the garlic and celery, and cook for a further 10 minutes until the celery is soft. Stir through the chorizo, chilli, and thyme, and cook for a minute. Add the sweet potatoes and cook for a few minutes, then add the peppers and let this cook gently for about 5 minutes, stirring so it doesn't stick.

2 Transfer everything to the slow cooker. Tip in the adzuki and kidney beans and the stock, stir, then cover with the lid and cook on auto/low for 8 hours or on high for 3 hours. Use a stick blender, or transfer in batches to a liquidizer, to blend until it is well combined but still retains some texture. Add a ladleful of hot water if it is too thick. Transfer the soup to a clean pan and heat through. Taste and season as needed, then ladle into warmed bowls and serve with torn tortilla bread, soured cream, a little grated Cheddar cheese, and a sprinkling of finely chopped parsley.

traditional method   PREP 10 MINS   COOK 1–1½ HRS

1 Heat the oil in a large heavy-based pan over a medium heat, add the onion, and cook for 3–4 minutes until soft. Season with salt and pepper, stir through the garlic and celery, and cook for a further 10 minutes until the celery is soft. Stir through the chorizo, chilli, and thyme, and cook for a minute. Add the sweet potatoes and cook for a few minutes, then add the peppers and let this cook gently for about 5 minutes, stirring so it doesn't stick.

2 Tip in the adzuki and kidney beans, add a little of the stock, increase the heat, and let the mixture simmer. Add the remaining stock, bring to the boil, then reduce to a simmer, partially cover with a lid, and cook for 45–60 minutes on a low heat. Check occasionally that it's not drying out, topping up with a little hot water if needed.

3 Use a stick blender, or transfer in batches to a liquidizer, to blend until it is well combined but still retains some texture. Add a ladleful of hot water if it is too thick. Transfer the soup to a clean pan and heat through. Taste and season as needed, then ladle into warmed bowls and serve with torn tortilla bread, soured cream, a little grated Cheddar cheese, and a sprinkling of finely chopped parsley.

A firm favourite with everyone, this soup tastes even better served the next day. Go easy on the salt when adding seasoning as the ham may be salty enough for most people's taste.

Pea, ham, and potato soup

⚙ **SERVES** 4–6   ❄ **FREEZE** UP TO 3 MONTHS

1.1kg (2½lb) unsmoked ham
1 bay leaf
1 tbsp olive oil
1 onion, finely chopped
salt and freshly ground black pepper
1 tbsp Dijon mustard
3 garlic cloves, finely chopped

2 sprigs of rosemary
handful of thyme, leaves only
900ml (1½ pints) hot beef stock for the slow cooker
   (1.2 litres/2 pints for the traditional method)
450g (1lb) frozen peas
3 potatoes, peeled and chopped into
   bite-sized pieces

in the slow cooker   🕒 **PREP** 15 MINS   **COOK** AUTO/LOW 8 HRS OR HIGH 4 HRS,
                                                    THEN **AUTO/LOW** 8 HRS OR **HIGH** 4 HRS

1 Preheat the slow cooker, if required. Sit the ham and bay leaf in the slow cooker and cover with 900ml (1½ pints) of water. Cover and cook on auto/low for 8 hours or on high for 4 hours, then remove the ham and set aside. Discard the stock, or strain and reserve a little to add to the soup.

2 Heat the oil in a large heavy-based pan over a medium heat, add the onion, and cook for 3–4 minutes until soft. Season with salt and pepper, then stir in the mustard, garlic, and herbs (reserve some thyme leaves for garnish). Add a little stock and bring to the boil, then tip in the peas (if you prefer them puréed, pulse them gently in a liquidizer or use a stick blender). Transfer to the slow cooker, add the remaining stock and the potatoes, cover, and cook on auto/low for 8 hours or on high for 4 hours. Remove any fat from the ham, chop into bite-sized pieces, and stir into the soup. Taste and season as needed. Garnish with the reserved thyme leaves and serve with wholemeal bread.

traditional method   🕒 **PREP** 15 MINS   **COOK** 2 HRS

1 Add the ham and bay leaf to a large pan, cover with 1.2 litres (2 pints) of water and bring to the boil. Partially cover, reduce to a simmer, and cook for about 1 hour or until the ham is cooked. Skim away any scum that comes to the surface of the pan as you go. Discard the stock, or strain and reserve a little to add to the soup. Set the ham aside until cool enough to handle.

2 Heat the oil in a large heavy-based pan over a medium heat, add the onion, and cook for 3–4 minutes until soft. Season with salt and pepper, then stir in the mustard, garlic, and herbs (reserve some thyme leaves for garnish). Add a little stock and bring to the boil, then tip in the peas and remaining stock. Bring to the boil, reduce to a simmer, and cook for 45 minutes, topping up with hot water as needed.

3 About 20 minutes before the end of the cooking time, bring a separate pan of water to the boil. Add the potatoes, bring back up to the boil, and then simmer for 12–15 minutes until soft. Drain and set aside. Remove the rosemary from the soup, then use a stick blender to gently purée the peas, or ladle them into a liquidizer and pulse a couple of times. Return them to the pan and stir in the potatoes. Remove any fat from the ham, chop into bite-sized pieces, and stir into the soup. Taste and season as needed. Garnish with the reserved thyme leaves and serve with wholemeal bread.

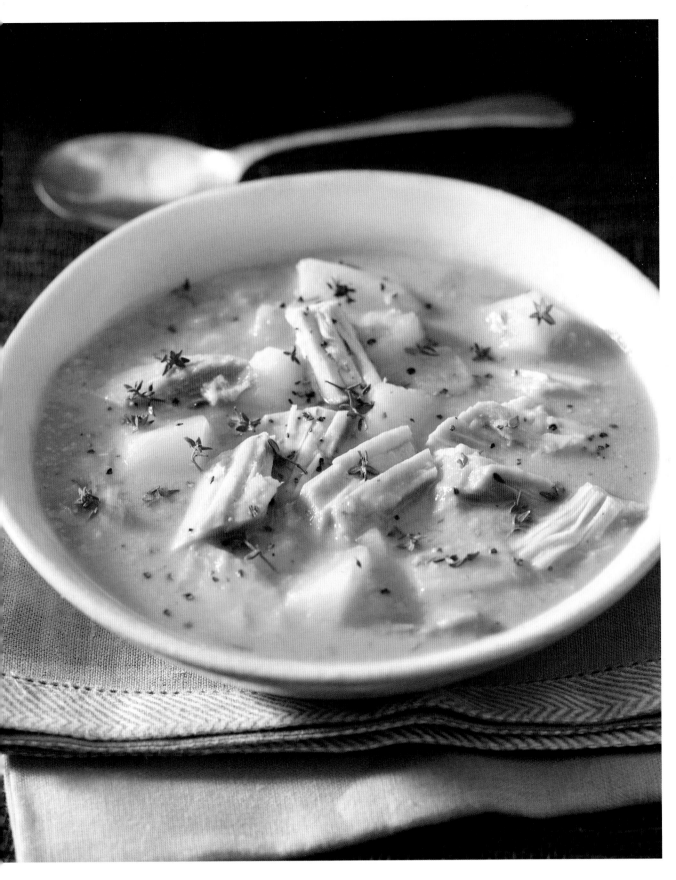

The subtle combinations of meaty monkfish, delicate haddock, aniseed fennel, and the light scent of saffron marry well. You could add some mussels or prawns, if you like.

Rich fish soup

SERVES 4–6   **FREEZE** UP TO 1 MONTH

1 tbsp olive oil
1 onion, finely chopped
salt and freshly ground black pepper
1 sprig of thyme
3 garlic cloves, finely chopped
1 fennel bulb, trimmed and finely chopped
1 red chilli, deseeded and finely chopped

250ml (9fl oz) dry white wine
2 x 400g cans chopped tomatoes
600ml (1 pint) hot light vegetable stock for the slow cooker (900ml/1½ pints for the traditional method)
pinch of saffron threads
200g (7oz) monkfish, cut into bite-sized pieces
200g (7oz) haddock loin, cut into bite-sized pieces

in the slow cooker   **PREP** 15 MINS   **COOK** 10 MINS PRECOOKING; AUTO/LOW 8 HRS OR **HIGH** 4 HRS

1 Preheat the slow cooker, if required. Heat the oil in a large heavy-based pan over a medium heat, add the onion, and cook for 3–4 minutes until soft. Season with salt and pepper and throw in the thyme. Add the garlic and fennel, and cook gently for a further 5 minutes until the fennel begins to soften.

2 Stir through the chilli and cook for 1 minute, then increase the heat, add the wine, and let it bubble for a minute. Transfer everything to the hot slow cooker, tip in the tomatoes and stock, and stir through the saffron. Cover with the lid and cook on auto/low for 8 hours or on high for 4 hours.

3 Use a stick blender to blend the soup until smooth, or transfer in batches to a liquidizer and blend until smooth and return to the hot slow cooker. Taste and season as needed, add the fish, put the lid back on, and leave for about 10 minutes or until the fish is opaque and cooked through. Ladle into warmed bowls and serve with white crusty bread. Garnish with chopped fennel fronds, if you like.

traditional method   **PREP** 15 MINS   **COOK** 1 HR

1 Heat the oil in a large heavy-based pan over a medium heat, add the onion, and cook for 3–4 minutes until soft. Season with salt and pepper and throw in the thyme. Add the garlic and fennel, and cook gently for a further 5 minutes until the fennel begins to soften.

2 Stir through the chilli and cook for 1 minute, then increase the heat, add the wine, let it bubble for a minute, and then tip in the canned tomatoes and stock. Add the saffron, bring to the boil, then reduce to a simmer and cook gently, partially covered with the lid, for about 45 minutes. Take care that the sauce doesn't dry out, topping it up with a little hot water if needed.

3 Use a stick blender to blend the soup until smooth, or transfer in batches to a liquidizer and blend until smooth, and return to a clean pan. Top up with a little hot water – you will probably need about 300ml (10fl oz) in total – and simmer gently. Taste and season as needed, add the fish, put the lid back on, and cook on a low heat for 6–10 minutes or until the fish is opaque and cooked through. Ladle into warmed bowls and serve with white crusty bread. Garnish with chopped fennel fronds, if you like.

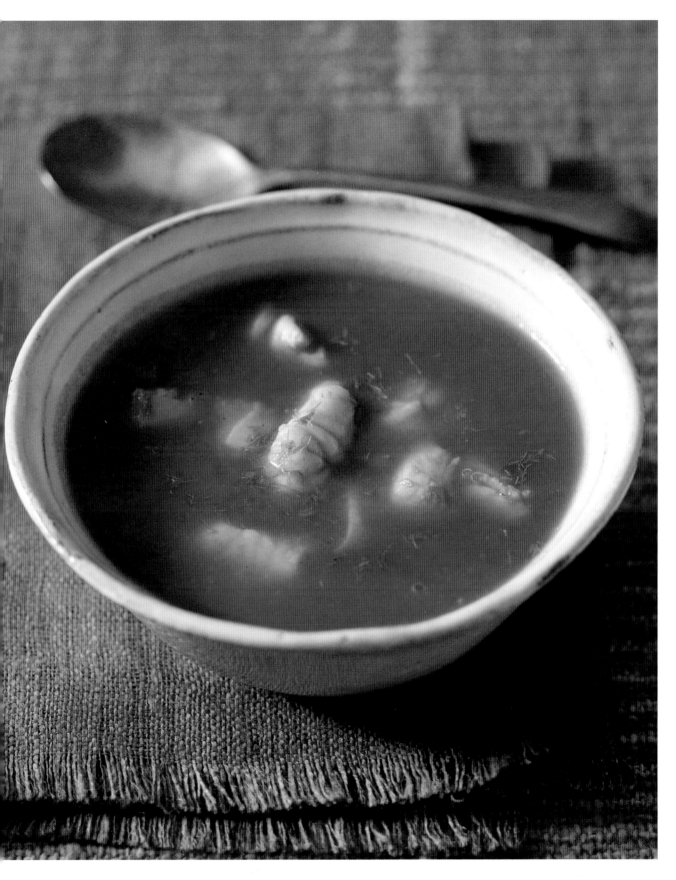

This velvety smooth soup can be made using pumpkin or butternut squash, depending on what is in season. The dried chilli flakes give it just the right kick to cut through the richness.

Pumpkin and ginger soup

SERVES 4–6 **FREEZE** UP TO 3 MONTHS

1 tbsp olive oil
1 onion, finely chopped
salt and freshly ground black pepper
3 garlic cloves, finely chopped
5cm (2in) piece of fresh root ginger,
  peeled and finely chopped
pinch of dried chilli flakes

1 small cinnamon stick
900g (2lb) pumpkin or butternut squash,
  peeled, deseeded, and diced
600ml (1 pint) hot vegetable stock for
  the slow cooker (900ml/1½ pints for the
  traditional method)

in the slow cooker
PREP 15 MINS **COOK** 15 MINS PRECOOKING;
AUTO/LOW 8 HRS OR HIGH 4 HRS

1 Preheat the slow cooker, if required. Heat the oil in a large heavy-based pan over a medium heat, add the onion, and cook for 3–4 minutes until soft. Season with salt and pepper, add the garlic, ginger, chilli flakes, and cinnamon stick, and cook for a few seconds before adding the pumpkin or squash (and a little more olive oil if needed) and stirring to coat.

2 Pour in a little of the stock, increase the heat, and scrape up the bits from the bottom of the pan. Transfer everything to the slow cooker. Add the remaining stock, cover with the lid, and cook on auto/low for 8 hours or on high for 4 hours.

3 Remove the cinnamon stick and use a stick blender to blend the soup until smooth, or transfer in batches to a liquidizer and blend until smooth. Transfer to a clean pan to heat through, taste, and season as required. Serve with some chunky wholemeal bread or some rye bread.

traditional method
PREP 15 MINS **COOK** 1 HR

1 Heat the oil in a large heavy-based pan over a medium heat, add the onion, and cook for 3–4 minutes until soft. Season with salt and pepper, add the garlic, ginger, chilli flakes, and cinnamon stick, and cook for a few seconds before adding the pumpkin or squash (and a little more olive oil if needed) and stirring to coat.

2 Pour in a little of the stock, increase the heat, and scrape up the bits from the bottom of the pan. Add the remaining stock, boil for 1 minute, then reduce the heat to barely a simmer, cover with the lid, and cook for about 45 minutes until the pumpkin is soft and the flavours have developed.

3 Remove the cinnamon stick and use a stick blender to blend the soup until smooth, or transfer in batches to a liquidizer and blend until smooth. Add a ladleful of hot water as you go if it is too thick. Transfer to a clean pan to heat through, taste, and season as required. Serve with some chunky wholemeal bread or some rye bread.

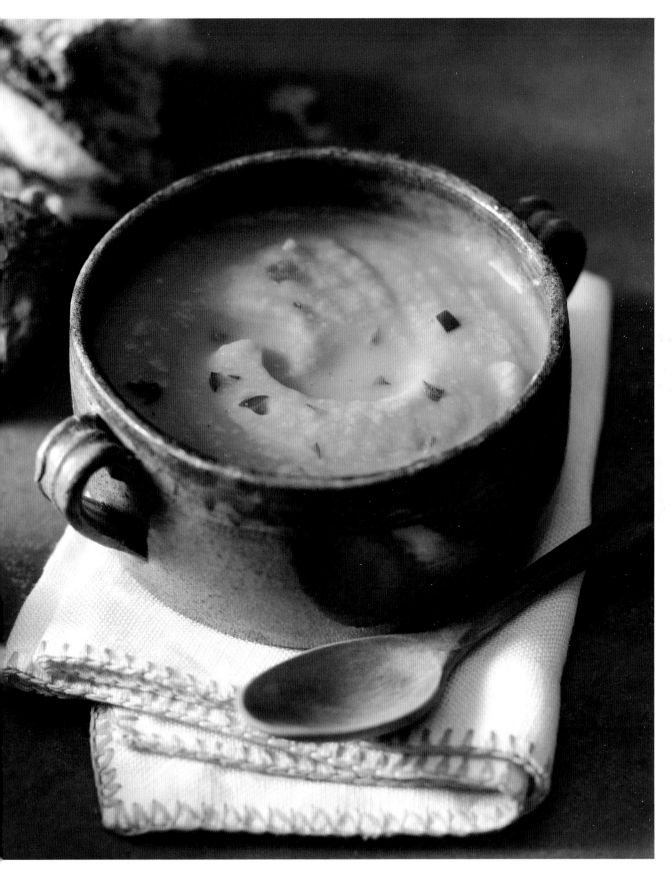

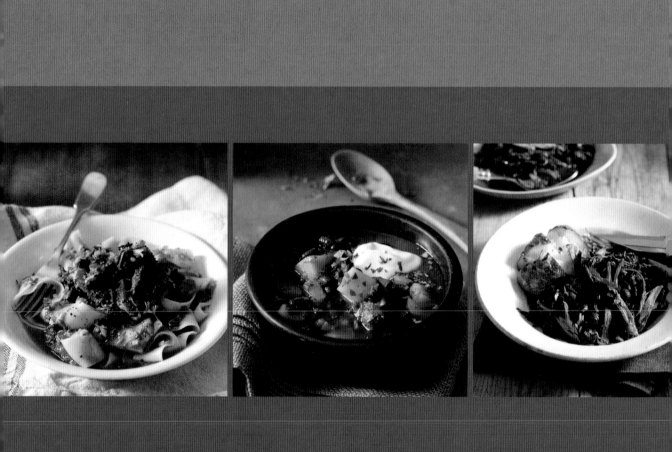

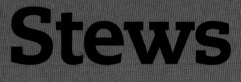

Stews

A colourful and gutsy dish, you could always add some spicy sausage or chorizo if you prefer a meaty meal. Black beans are also called turtle beans and need soaking overnight.

Brazilian black bean and pumpkin stew

⊙ **SERVES** 4–6 ❄ **FREEZE** UP TO 3 MONTHS ♡ **HEALTHY**

325g (11oz) dried black beans, soaked
  overnight and drained
1 tbsp olive oil
1 onion, finely chopped
salt and freshly ground black pepper
3 garlic cloves, finely chopped
1 small pumpkin or butternut squash, peeled,
  deseeded, and diced

2 red peppers, deseeded and diced
2 x 400g cans chopped tomatoes
1 small green chilli, deseeded and diced
600ml (1 pint) hot vegetable stock for the slow
  cooker (900ml/1½ pints for the traditional method)
1 mango, peeled, stone removed, and diced
bunch of coriander, chopped

in the slow cooker 🕐 **PREP** 25 MINS, PLUS SOAKING **COOK** 10 MINS PRECOOKING;
AUTO/LOW 6–8 HRS

1 Preheat the slow cooker, if required. Put the beans in a large heavy-based pan and cover with water. Bring to the boil, and then drain the beans and set aside.

2 Dry the pan and heat the oil in it over a medium heat, add the onion, and cook for 3–4 minutes until soft. Season with salt and pepper, stir in the garlic, and cook for 1–2 minutes until soft. Stir in the pumpkin or butternut squash and also cook for about a minute.

3 Transfer everything to the slow cooker and add the beans, red peppers, tomatoes, and chilli together with the stock. Season well, cover with the lid, and cook on auto/low for 6–8 hours. Taste and season, if necessary, then stir through the mango and coriander. Serve with some soured cream and rice on the side.

traditional method 🕐 **PREP** 25 MINS, PLUS SOAKING **COOK** 2½–3 HRS

1 Preheat the oven to 160°C (325°F/Gas 3). Put the beans in a large heavy-based pan and cover with water. Bring to the boil, then reduce to a simmer, partially cover with the lid, and cook on a low heat for 1 hour. Drain and set aside.

2 Heat the oil in a large heavy-based pan over a medium heat, add the onion, and cook for 3–4 minutes until soft. Season with salt and pepper, stir in the garlic, and cook for 1–2 minutes until soft. Stir in the pumpkin or butternut squash, red peppers, tomatoes, and chilli.

3 Add the beans, pour over the stock, and bring to the boil. Then reduce to a simmer, cover with the lid and put in the oven for 1½–2 hours. Taste and season, if necessary, then stir through the mango and coriander. Serve with some soured cream and rice on the side.

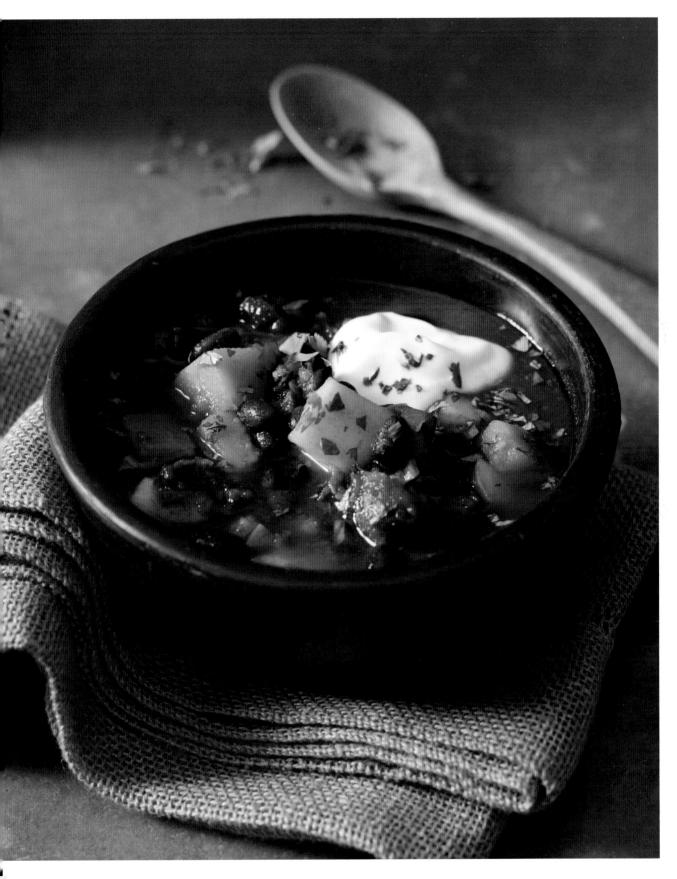

This combination of rich pork and salty clams – and, indeed, any pork with shellfish – has been enjoyed for centuries in Portugal. A squeeze of lemon at the end brings out the flavours.

Pork and clam cataplana

SERVES 4 **FREEZE** UP TO 1 MONTH, WITHOUT THE CLAMS **HEALTHY**

900g (2lb) pork tenderloin, cut into 2.5cm (1in) cubes
2 tbsp olive oil
1 large onion, thinly sliced
2 garlic cloves, finely chopped
400g can whole tomatoes
1 tbsp tomato purée
dash of Tabasco sauce (or more to taste)
1kg (2¼lb) clams, such as amandes, scrubbed
  (discard any that do not close when tapped)
bunch of parsley, leaves chopped

FOR THE MARINADE
2 garlic cloves, finely chopped
1 bay leaf
1½ tbsp paprika
1 tbsp olive oil
375ml (13fl oz) dry white wine
pinch of freshly ground black pepper

in the slow cooker
PREP 20 MINS, PLUS MARINATING
COOK 30 MINS PRECOOKING; **AUTO/LOW** 6–8 HRS OR **HIGH** 3–4 HRS

1 To make the marinade, put all the ingredients into a bowl and whisk to combine. Add the pork and mix well. Cover and refrigerate for 2 hours, or 12 hours if time permits, stirring occasionally. Preheat the slow cooker, if required. Lift the meat from the marinade with a slotted spoon and pat dry with kitchen paper. Reserve the marinade. Heat the oil in a large flameproof casserole over a medium-high heat. Add the pork, in batches, and brown well on all sides. Transfer to a bowl and set aside.

2 Reduce the heat and add the onion and garlic to the casserole. Cover and cook very gently for about 15 minutes, until the onion is very soft and brown. Add the tomatoes, tomato purée, Tabasco, and pork. Pour in the marinade and stir. Transfer everything to the slow cooker, cover with the lid, and cook on auto/low for 6–8 hours or on high for 3–4 hours. Add the clams for the last 20 minutes of cooking, or until all the clams are open (discard any that do not open). Transfer to a warmed serving bowl, remove the bay leaf, sprinkle with the parsley, and serve with lemon wedges on the side.

traditional method
PREP 20 MINS, PLUS MARINATING **COOK** 2¼–2½ HRS

1 To make the marinade, put all the ingredients into a bowl and whisk to combine. Add the pork and mix well. Cover and refrigerate for 2 hours, or 12 hours if time permits, stirring occasionally. Preheat the oven to 180°C (350°F/Gas 4). Lift the meat from the marinade with a slotted spoon and pat dry with kitchen paper. Reserve the marinade. Heat the oil in a large flameproof casserole over a medium-high heat. Add the pork, in batches, and brown well on all sides. Transfer to a bowl and set aside.

2 Reduce the heat and add the onion and garlic to the casserole. Cover and cook very gently for about 15 minutes, until the onion is very soft and brown. Add the tomatoes, tomato purée, Tabasco, and pork. Pour in the marinade and stir. Cover with the lid and cook in the oven for 1½–1¾ hours, until tender when pierced. Check occasionally that it's not drying out, topping up with a little hot water if needed. Arrange the clams on top of the pork, cover with the lid, and cook in the oven for 15–20 minutes longer until the clams open (discard any that do not open). Transfer to a warmed serving bowl, remove the bay leaf, sprinkle with the parsley, and serve with lemon wedges on the side.

This is a filling one-pot meal, known as *Cocido* in Spain. Vary the vegetables, if you wish – turnip, green beans, or even pumpkin are all delicious. Chickpeas are a must for this dish.

Spanish stew

SERVES 6

3 tbsp olive oil
2 small onions, quartered
2 garlic cloves, sliced
2 slices pork belly, about 550g (1¼lb), cut into large chunks
4 chicken thighs, about 600g (1lb 5oz) total weight
115g (4oz) beef braising steak, cut into bite-sized pieces
115g (4oz) tocino or smoked streaky bacon, cut into bite-sized pieces
4 small pork spare ribs, 150g (5½oz) total weight

100ml (3½fl oz) white wine
115g (4oz) chorizo, chopped into 4 pieces
115g (4oz) morcilla (Spanish black pudding) (optional)
1 bay leaf
salt and freshly ground black pepper
6 small waxy potatoes, chopped into large chunks
3 carrots, peeled and chopped into large chunks
400g can chickpeas, drained
½ Savoy cabbage or green cabbage heart, cored and quartered
3 tbsp chopped parsley, to serve

in the slow cooker   **PREP** 35 MINS   **COOK** 30 MINS PRECOOKING; **AUTO/LOW** 6–8 HRS

1 Preheat the slow cooker, if required. Heat 1 tbsp of the oil in a large flameproof casserole over a medium heat, add the onions and garlic, and cook for 10 minutes, stirring occasionally. Transfer to the slow cooker. Heat the remaining oil in the casserole and cook the pork, chicken, beef, tocino or bacon, and spare ribs, in batches, until lightly browned on all sides. Also transfer to the slow cooker.

2 Pour the wine into the casserole and reduce by half over a high heat. Add to the slow cooker along with the chorizo, morcilla, if using, and bay leaf, season with salt and pepper, then pour in enough hot water to cover. Cover with the lid and cook on auto/low for 6–8 hours, adding the potatoes, carrots, chickpeas, and cabbage for the last hour of cooking. Remove the bay leaf, bones, and chicken skin from the stew. Divide the meat and vegetables between warmed serving plates. Add a few spoonfuls of the hot broth and sprinkle with parsley. Serve with crusty bread.

traditional method   **PREP** 35 MINS   **COOK** 2¾ HRS

1 Heat 1 tbsp of the oil in a large flameproof casserole over a medium heat, add the onions and garlic, and cook for 10 minutes, stirring occasionally. Remove and set aside in a bowl. Heat the remaining oil in the casserole and cook the pork, chicken, beef, tocino, and spare ribs, in batches, until lightly browned on all sides. Transfer to the bowl with the onions.

2 Pour the wine into the casserole and reduce by half over a high heat. Add the chorizo, morcilla, if using, and bay leaf together with the onions and browned meat. Season with salt and pepper, then pour in enough cold water to cover. Bring to the boil, then reduce the heat and simmer, covered, for 1½ hours. Add the potatoes and carrots to the casserole, continue to cook for 15 minutes, then add the chickpeas and cabbage and cook for a further 15 minutes. Remove the bay leaf, bones, and chicken skin from the stew. Divide the meat and vegetables between warmed serving plates. Add a few spoonfuls of the hot broth and sprinkle with parsley. Serve with crusty bread.

Slow-cooked sweet cabbage is the perfect complement to ham, and with the addition of spices and dried fruit, the humble piece of meat is transformed. Ham hocks are also known as knuckles.

Ham hock with red cabbage

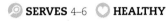 **SERVES** 4–6 **HEALTHY**

2 ham hocks, about 1.35kg (3lb) each
1 red cabbage, cored and finely shredded
2 onions, sliced
4 garlic cloves, finely chopped
few sprigs of thyme
60g (2oz) raisins

pinch of freshly grated nutmeg
pinch of ground cinnamon
150ml (5fl oz) white wine vinegar for the slow cooker
  (300ml/10fl oz for the traditional method)
600ml (1 pint) hot vegetable stock, for both methods
salt and freshly ground black pepper

in the slow cooker **PREP** 20 MINS **COOK** AUTO/LOW 6–8 HRS, THEN AUTO/LOW 6–8 HRS

1 Preheat the slow cooker, if required. Put the ham hocks in the pot and cover with water so that the cooker is three-quarters full. Cover with the lid and cook on auto/low for 6–8 hours.

2 Remove the hams and reserve the cooking liquid, if you wish to use it instead of the vegetable stock (it can be salty). When the hams are cool enough to handle, remove the skin and discard, then sit the hams back in the slow cooker. Add all the other ingredients, using either the stock or the cooking liquid, and season with salt and pepper. Cover with the lid and cook on auto/low for 6–8 hours. Remove the hams, shred the meat, and stir it into the slow cooker. Serve with baked or roast potatoes.

traditional method **PREP** 20 MINS **COOK** 3 HRS

1 Preheat the oven to 160°C (325°F/Gas 3). Sit the ham hocks in a large heavy-based pan and cover with water. Bring to the boil, then reduce to a simmer, partially cover, and cook gently for 1 hour. Remove the hams and reserve the stock, if you wish to use it instead of the vegetable stock (it can be salty). When the hams are cool enough to handle, remove the skin and discard, then sit the hams in a large flameproof casserole.

2 Add all the other ingredients to the casserole, using either the stock or the cooking liquid, and tuck the hams in neatly. Season with salt and pepper, cover, and put in the oven for 2 hours. Check occasionally that it's not drying out, topping up with a little hot water if necessary. Remove the hams, shred the meat, and stir it into the casserole. Serve with baked or roast potatoes.

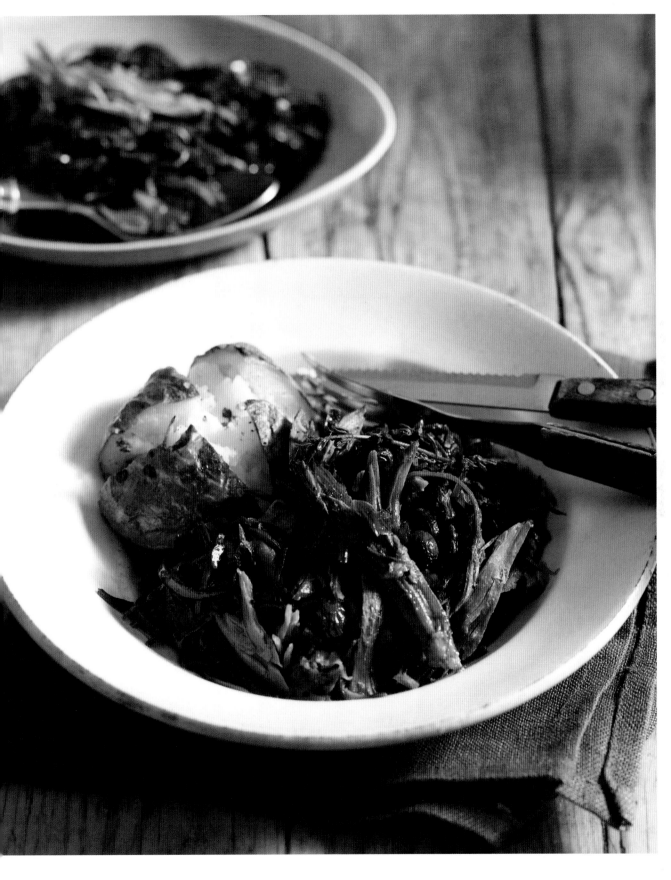

Barley is a grain that used to be overlooked, but it has made a well-deserved comeback due to its ability to add body and earthy flavour to all sorts of dishes. For a treat, use wild mushrooms, too.

Beef with barley and mushrooms

SERVES 4–6 **FREEZE** UP TO 3 MONTHS

3 tbsp vegetable oil
1kg (2¼lb) braising steak, cut into 5cm (2in) pieces
450g (1lb) onions, thinly sliced
salt and freshly ground black pepper
1 bouquet garni, made with 5–6 parsley sprigs,
  2–3 thyme sprigs, and 1 bay leaf
700ml (1 pint 3½fl oz) hot beef stock for the slow
  cooker (1 litre/1¾ pints for the traditional method)

225g (8oz) carrots, sliced
2 celery sticks, sliced
150g (5½oz) pearl barley
500g (1lb 2oz) mushrooms, trimmed and sliced
2–3 sprigs of parsley, leaves finely chopped, to serve

in the slow cooker **PREP** 30 MINS **COOK** 20 MINS PRECOOKING;
AUTO/LOW 6–8 HRS OR **HIGH** 3–4 HRS

1 Preheat the slow cooker, if required. Heat the oil in a large flameproof casserole over a medium-high heat, add the beef (in batches, if necessary) and cook for about 5 minutes until well browned. Remove and set aside.

2 Reduce the heat to medium, add the onions and a little salt and pepper, and cook for 5–7 minutes until lightly browned. Return the beef and add the bouquet garni and more seasoning. Pour in the stock, stir, and then add the carrots, celery, and barley. Transfer everything to the slow cooker, cover, and cook on auto/low for 6–8 hours or on high for 3–4 hours. Add the mushrooms for the last 20 minutes of cooking.

3 Discard the bouquet garni and taste the stew for seasoning, adding more if needed. Serve in warmed bowls, sprinkled with the parsley and with crusty bread on the side.

traditional method **PREP** 30 MINS **COOK** 2¼–2½ HRS

1 Preheat the oven to 180°C (350°F/Gas 4). Heat the oil in a large flameproof casserole over a medium-high heat, add the beef (in batches, if necessary) and cook for about 5 minutes until well browned. Remove and set aside.

2 Reduce the heat to medium, add the onions and a little salt and pepper, and cook for 5–7 minutes until lightly browned. Return the beef and add the bouquet garni and more seasoning. Pour in the stock and stir. Cover with the lid and put in the oven for 1½ hours, stirring occasionally. Then add the carrots, celery, and barley, together with more hot water, if necessary, to keep the casserole moist. Cover, and continue to cook for a further 40–45 minutes until the meat and vegetables are tender when pierced. The barley should be tender but still slightly chewy. About 20 minutes before the end of cooking, stir in the mushrooms.

3 Discard the bouquet garni and taste the stew for seasoning, adding more if needed. Serve in warmed bowls, sprinkled with the parsley and with crusty bread on the side.

In this dish, salt cod is tender and fragrant with the classic Spanish aromas of garlic, bay leaves, and saffron. If you can't get salt cod, use a white fish and add it in for the last 15 minutes of cooking.

Salt cod braised with vegetables

SERVES 4 **HEALTHY**

800g (1¾lb) thick-cut salt cod, or fresh white fish
  such as sustainable cod, haddock, or halibut
3 tbsp olive oil
1 onion, finely diced
2 leeks, trimmed and white parts finely sliced
3 garlic cloves, finely chopped
3 tomatoes, skinned and chopped

500g (1lb 2oz) potatoes, diced
salt and freshly ground black pepper
2 bay leaves
large pinch of saffron threads
120ml (4fl oz) dry white wine
2 tbsp chopped parsley, to serve

in the slow cooker **PREP** 20 MINS, PLUS SOAKING **COOK** 10 MINS PRECOOKING; AUTO/LOW 6–8 HRS OR **HIGH** 3–4 HRS

1 If using the salt cod, soak the pieces of cod in enough cold water to cover them for at least 24 hours, changing the water 2–3 times to remove the saltiness of the brine. Drain and cut the fish into 4 pieces, then pat dry with kitchen paper. If using the fresh fish, simply cut the fish into 4 pieces.

2 Preheat the slow cooker, if required. Heat the oil in a large heavy-based pan over a medium heat, add the onion and leeks, and cook for about 5 minutes until soft. Add the garlic and tomatoes and cook for a further 2 minutes, stirring. Add the potatoes, seasoning, bay leaves, and saffron.

3 Transfer everything to the slow cooker, then pour in the wine and 100ml (3½fl oz) of water. Cover with the lid and cook on auto/low for 6–8 hours or on high for 3–4 hours. Sit the salt cod, skin-side up, on top of the vegetables for the last hour of cooking. Ladle into warmed bowls, sprinkle with the parsley, and serve with a crisp mixed salad and some crusty bread.

traditional method **PREP** 20 MINS, PLUS SOAKING **COOK** 40 MINS

1 If using the salt cod, soak the pieces of cod in enough cold water to cover them for at least 24 hours, changing the water 2–3 times to remove the saltiness of the brine. Drain and cut the fish into 4 pieces, then pat dry with kitchen paper. If using the fresh fish, simply cut the fish into 4 pieces.

2 Heat the oil in a large heavy-based pan over a medium heat, add the onion and leeks, and cook for about 5 minutes until soft. Add the garlic and tomatoes and cook for a further 2 minutes, stirring. Add the potatoes, seasoning, bay leaves, and saffron.

3 Pour in the wine and 250ml (9fl oz) water and sit the cod, skin-side up, on top of the vegetables. Bring gently to a simmer and cook for 25–30 minutes until the fish is opaque and cooked through. Shake the pan once or twice every 5 minutes to help release gelatine from the fish, to thicken the sauce. Ladle into warmed bowls, sprinkle with the parsley, and serve with a crisp mixed salad and some crusty bread.

In Italy, this dish is called *alla cacciatora*, meaning "hunter's style". Chicory, with its slight bitterness, makes a flavoursome addition and must be added towards the end of cooking.

Hunter's chicken stew

⊙ **SERVES** 4 ✲ **FREEZE** UP TO 3 MONTHS, WITHOUT THE CHICORY

1.5kg (3lb 3oz) chicken, jointed into 8 pieces
salt and freshly ground black pepper
4 tbsp olive oil
1 onion, chopped
4 garlic cloves, finely chopped
1 sprig of rosemary

1 bay leaf
4 tbsp dry white wine
120ml (4fl oz) hot chicken stock, for both methods
2 heads of chicory (also known as Belgian endive), trimmed, leaves separated, and roughly chopped

in the slow cooker 🕐 **PREP** 15 MINS **COOK** 30 MINS PRECOOKING; AUTO/LOW 5–6 HRS OR HIGH 3–4 HRS

1 Preheat the slow cooker, if required. Season the chicken all over with salt and pepper. Heat half the oil in a large flameproof casserole over a medium heat, add the thighs and drumsticks, skin-side down, and cook for about 5 minutes until they begin to brown. Add the breast pieces and cook gently for 10–15 minutes until very brown. Turn and brown the other side. Lower the heat.

2 Add the onion and garlic, stir, and continue cooking gently for 3–4 minutes until they are soft. Season with salt and pepper, then stir in the rosemary, bay leaf, wine, and stock, and bring to the boil. Transfer everything to the slow cooker, cover with the lid, and cook on auto/low for 5–6 hours or on high for 3–4 hours.

3 Add the chicory for the last 15 minutes of cooking. Discard the bay leaf and rosemary from the sauce, taste, and add seasoning if needed. Spoon out into warmed bowls and serve with crusty bread.

traditional method 🕐 **PREP** 20–25 MINS **COOK** 45–60 MINS

1 Season the chicken all over with salt and pepper. Heat half the oil in a large flameproof casserole over a medium heat, add the thighs and drumsticks, skin-side down, and cook for about 5 minutes until they begin to brown. Add the breast pieces and cook gently for 10–15 minutes until very brown. Turn and brown the other side. Lower the heat.

2 Add the onion and garlic, stir, and continue cooking gently for 3–4 minutes until they are soft. Season with salt and pepper, then stir in the rosemary, bay leaf, wine, and stock. Cover and simmer for 15–20 minutes until tender.

3 Add the chicory for the last 5 minutes of cooking, return the lid, and cook gently until it has just softened. Discard the bay leaf and rosemary from the sauce, taste, and add seasoning if needed. Spoon out into warmed bowls and serve with crusty bread.

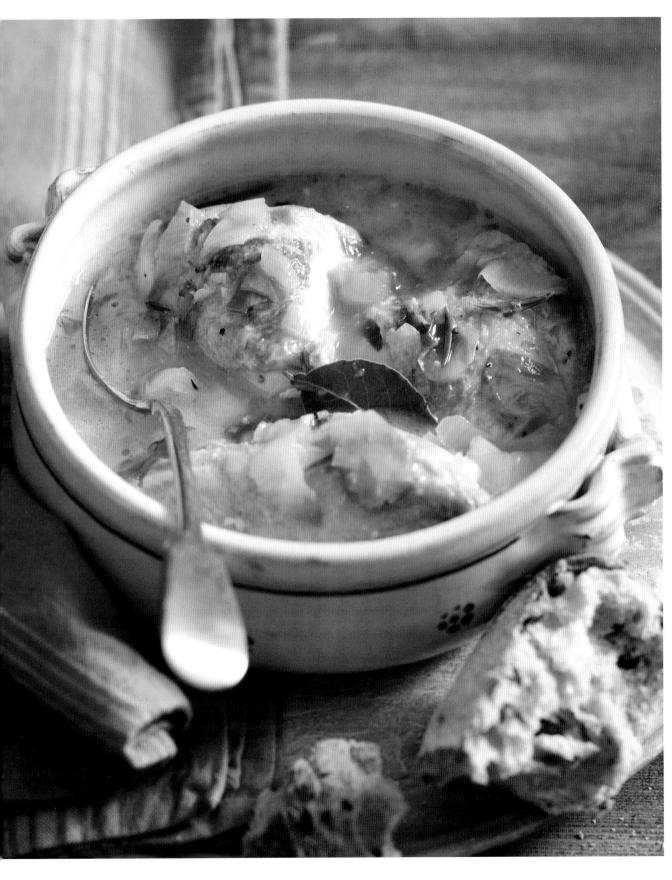

Olives, feta cheese, and thyme are all synonymous with Greek cuisine, and here they are combined with a succulent leg of lamb. The feta adds a fabulous saltiness to the finished dish.

Stuffed lamb, Greek style

SERVES 4–6

1 leg of lamb, boned and butterflied
   (about 1.8kg/4lb after boning – ask your butcher
   to do this), or use a boneless shoulder
salt and freshly ground black pepper
2 tbsp olive oil
1 tbsp dried oregano
2 red peppers, deseeded and finely chopped

60g (2oz) stoned black olives, finely chopped
175g (6oz) feta cheese, finely chopped
3 red onions, roughly chopped
4–6 tomatoes, roughly chopped
450ml (15fl oz) red wine
few sprigs of thyme

in the slow cooker   PREP 30 MINS   COOK 10 MINS PRECOOKING; AUTO/LOW 8 HRS

1 Preheat the slow cooker, if required. Lay the lamb out flat and season well. Rub both sides all over with the oil and oregano. Cover one side of the lamb with the red peppers, then the olives, and then the feta. Starting from one end, roll up the lamb, tucking in any loose pieces to neaten it. Tie it up with butcher's string so it is secure.

2 Heat a large flameproof casserole over a medium heat, add the lamb, and cook for 4–6 minutes on each side until it begins to colour. Transfer the lamb to the slow cooker and add the onions, tomatoes, and wine. Season and add the thyme, cover with the lid, and cook on auto/low for 8 hours.

3 Remove the meat from the slow cooker, cover loosely with foil, and leave to rest for 15 minutes. Remove the string and carve into slices. Serve with some of the sauce, together with baby roast potatoes with rosemary, and some wilted spinach.

traditional method   PREP 30 MINS   COOK 2¼–2¾ HRS

1 Preheat the oven to 160°C (325°F/Gas 3). Lay the lamb out flat and season well. Rub both sides all over with the oil and oregano. Cover one side of the lamb with the red peppers, then the olives, and then the feta. Starting from one end, roll up the lamb, tucking in any loose pieces to neaten it. Tie it up with butcher's string so it is secure.

2 Heat a large flameproof casserole over a medium heat, add the lamb, and cook for 4–6 minutes on each side until it begins to colour. Throw in the red onions and tomatoes and cook for a minute more, then pour in the wine. Bring to the boil, then reduce to a simmer and add some seasoning and the thyme. Cover with the lid and put in the oven for 2–2½ hours or until cooked to your liking. Check occasionally that it's not drying out, topping up with a little hot water if needed.

3 Remove from the oven, cover the meat loosely with foil, and leave to rest for 15 minutes. Remove the string and carve into slices. Serve with some of the sauce, together with baby roast potatoes with rosemary, and some wilted spinach.

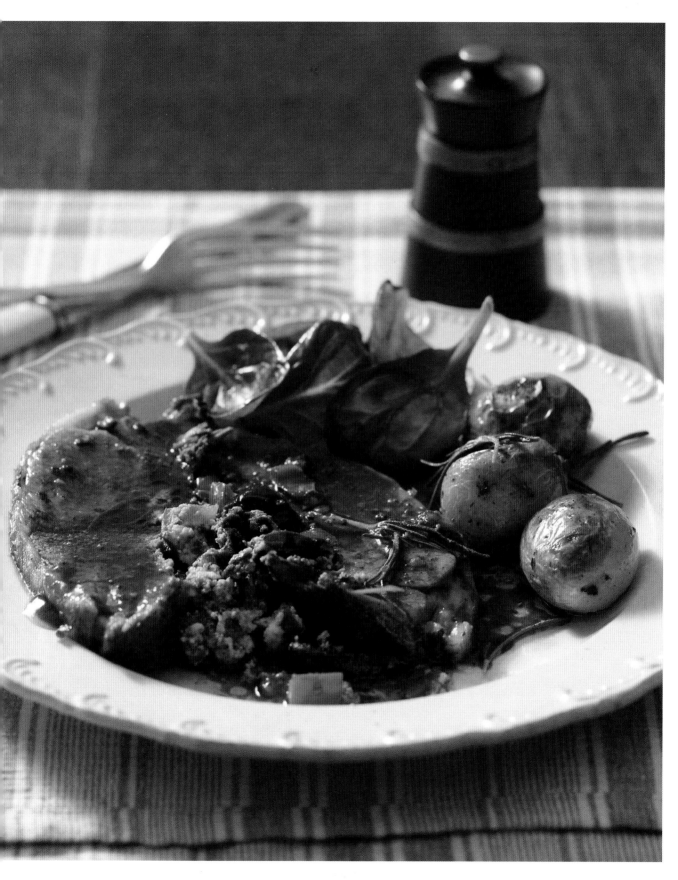

There is plenty of vibrant colour and a lot of heat in this vegetable dish. This is good on its own or with plain boiled rice and, to ring the changes, you may wish to add some chorizo or chicken.

Jamaican corn stew

SERVES 4–6

2 tbsp olive oil
2 onions, finely chopped
salt and freshly ground black pepper
3 garlic cloves, finely chopped
1 tsp cayenne pepper
3 sweetcorn cobs, cut into slices about
  1cm (½in) thick
2 red peppers, deseeded and roughly chopped

3 sweet potatoes, peeled and diced
175g (6oz) yellow split peas
150ml (5fl oz) hot vegetable stock for the slow
  cooker (300ml/10fl oz for the traditional method)
400ml can coconut milk
small handful of thyme
1 Scotch bonnet chilli, left whole

in the slow cooker **PREP** 20 MINS **COOK** 10 MINS PRECOOKING;
AUTO/LOW 6–8 HRS OR **HIGH** 3–4 HRS

1 Preheat the slow cooker, if required. Heat the oil in a large heavy-based pan over a medium heat, add the onions, and cook for 3–4 minutes until soft. Season with salt and pepper, then stir through the garlic and cayenne pepper, and cook for 1 minute. Add the sweetcorn, peppers, and sweet potatoes and turn so it is all coated evenly. Then stir through the split peas and a little of the stock.

2 Transfer the mixture to the slow cooker. Pour in the coconut milk and the remaining stock. Add seasoning, the thyme, and the Scotch bonnet, then stir, cover with the lid, and cook on auto/low for 6–8 hours or on high for 3–4 hours.

3 Remove the Scotch bonnet, taste, and season as required. Ladle into warmed bowls and serve with rice and some lime wedges on the side.

traditional method **PREP** 20 MINS **COOK** 1½–2 HRS

1 Preheat the oven to 160°C (325°F/Gas 3). Heat the oil in a large flameproof casserole over a medium heat, add the onions, and cook for 3–4 minutes until soft. Season with salt and pepper, then stir through the garlic and cayenne pepper, and cook for 1 minute. Add the sweetcorn, peppers, and sweet potatoes and turn so it is all coated evenly. Then stir through the split peas and a little of the stock.

2 Bring to the boil, then add the remaining stock and coconut milk. Bring back to the boil, reduce to a simmer, season, and add the thyme and the Scotch bonnet. Cover and put in the oven to cook for 1½–2 hours. Check occasionally that it's not drying out, topping up with a little hot water if needed.

3 Remove the Scotch bonnet, taste, and season as required. Ladle into warmed bowls and serve with rice and some lime wedges on the side.

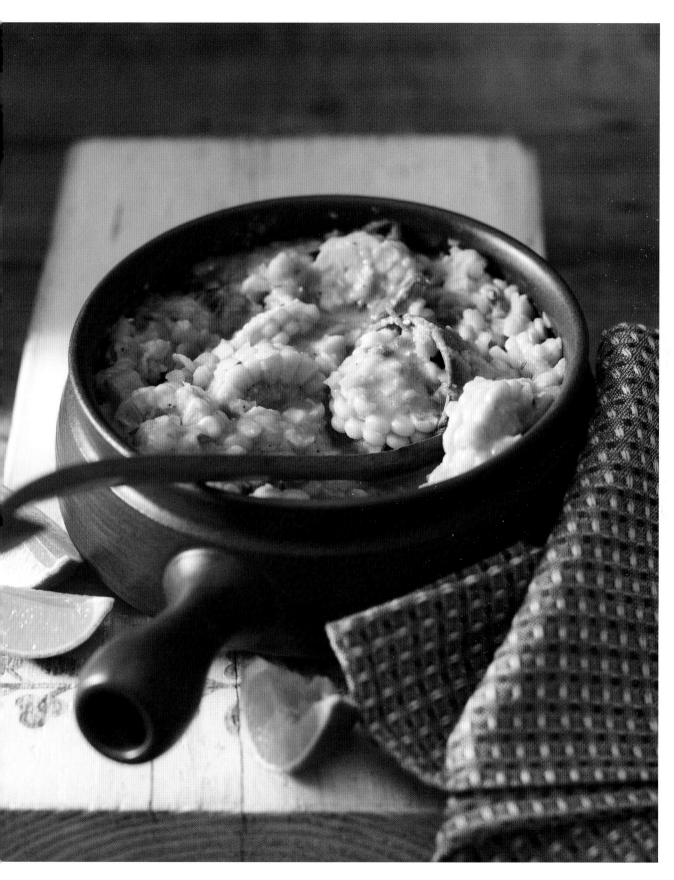

Chianti is the wine of Tuscany, but you can use any good-quality, full-bodied red wine. This dish benefits from being made ahead and kept in the refrigerator; its flavours will mellow.

Peppery Tuscan beef

SERVES 4–6 **FREEZE** UP TO 3 MONTHS

2 tbsp freshly ground black pepper
200ml (7fl oz) olive oil, plus 3 tbsp for cooking
1.1kg (2½lb) braising steak, cut into 5cm (2in) cubes
125g (4½oz) pancetta lardons
1 large onion, chopped
5 garlic cloves, finely chopped

400g can chopped tomatoes
2 bay leaves
3–4 sprigs of sage, leaves chopped
250ml (9fl oz) hot beef stock, for both methods
300ml (10fl oz) red wine for the slow cooker
    (500ml/16fl oz for the traditional method)

in the slow cooker **PREP** 20 MINS, PLUS MARINATING **COOK** 20 MINS PRECOOKING; AUTO/LOW 8 HRS

1 In a large bowl, combine 1 tbsp of the black pepper with the oil. Add the beef and stir until well coated. Cover with cling film and refrigerate, stirring occasionally, for 8–12 hours.

2 Preheat the slow cooker, if required. Remove the beef from the marinade and pat dry with kitchen paper. Heat the cooking oil in a large flameproof casserole over a high heat, add the meat (in batches, if necessary), and cook for 3–5 minutes until browned on all sides. Remove and set aside. Reduce the heat to medium, add the lardons, and cook, stirring occasionally, for 2–3 minutes, until the fat has rendered. Add the onion and cook for 3–4 minutes until soft. Return the beef and add the garlic, tomatoes, bay leaves, sage, stock, and wine, together with the remaining pepper. Bring to the boil, then transfer everything to the slow cooker, cover with the lid, and cook on auto/low for 8 hours.

3 Discard the bay leaves, taste, and add seasoning if needed. Serve with some greens, such as Savoy cabbage or broccoli, and Italian-style cubed roast potatoes and rosemary.

traditional method **PREP** 20 MINS, PLUS MARINATING **COOK** 2–2½ HRS

1 In a large bowl, combine 1 tbsp of the black pepper with the oil. Add the beef and stir until well coated. Cover with cling film and refrigerate, stirring occasionally, for 8–12 hours.

2 Remove the beef from the marinade and pat dry with kitchen paper. Heat the cooking oil in a large flameproof casserole over a high heat, add the meat (in batches, if necessary), and cook for 3–5 minutes until browned on all sides. Remove and set aside. Reduce the heat to medium, add the lardons, and cook, stirring occasionally, for 2–3 minutes, until the fat has rendered. Add the onion and cook for 3–4 minutes until soft. Return the beef and add the garlic, tomatoes, bay leaves, sage, stock, and wine, together with the remaining pepper. Bring to the boil, cover, reduce the heat, and leave to simmer for 1¾–2 hours until very tender, stirring occasionally. During cooking, add more hot water if the stew seems dry. The beef is ready when it is tender enough to crush in your fingers.

3 Discard the bay leaves, taste, and add seasoning if needed. Serve with some greens, such as Savoy cabbage or broccoli, and Italian-style cubed roast potatoes and rosemary.

In Mexico, chorizo is made with fresh pork, but in Spain, the pork is smoked first for even more flavour. Chorizo works its magic as it cooks and gives the sauce a rich, deep flavour.

Chicken with chorizo

SERVES 4 **FREEZE** UP TO 1 MONTH

2 tbsp olive oil
4 skinless chicken legs
250g (9oz) chorizo, chopped into bite-sized pieces
1 red onion, thinly sliced
1 tsp ground coriander
1 tsp chopped thyme leaves
1 red pepper, deseeded and chopped
1 yellow pepper, deseeded and chopped

1 courgette, trimmed and sliced
2 garlic cloves, crushed
400g can chopped tomatoes
100ml (3½fl oz) hot chicken stock for the slow cooker (200ml/7fl oz for the traditional method)
60ml (2fl oz) dry sherry
freshly ground black pepper

in the slow cooker

PREP 10 MINS **COOK** 20 MINS PRECOOKING; **AUTO/LOW** 6–8 HRS OR **HIGH** 3–4 HRS

1 Preheat the slow cooker, if required. Heat the oil in a large flameproof casserole over a medium-high heat, add the chicken, and fry for 5–8 minutes, turning frequently, until evenly browned. Remove and set aside. Then add the chorizo to the casserole and cook for 2–3 minutes until lightly browned, stirring frequently. Also remove and set aside.

2 Reduce the heat to medium, add the onion to the casserole, and cook for 3–4 minutes until soft. Add the coriander, cook for 1 minute, and then add the thyme, peppers, courgette, and garlic and cook for 5 minutes. Add the tomatoes, stock, and sherry. Season with black pepper, if needed, and bring to the boil. Transfer everything to the slow cooker, including the chicken and chorizo. Cover with the lid and cook on auto/low for 6–8 hours or on high for 3–4 hours. Serve with mashed sweet potatoes and peas.

traditional method

PREP 10 MINS **COOK** 1 HR

1 Preheat the oven to 180°C (350°F/Gas 4). Heat the oil in a large flameproof casserole over a medium-high heat, add the chicken, and fry for 5–8 minutes, turning frequently, until evenly browned. Remove and set aside. Then add the chorizo to the casserole and cook for 2–3 minutes until lightly browned, stirring frequently. Also remove and set aside.

2 Reduce the heat to medium, add the onion to the casserole, and cook for 3–4 minutes until soft. Add the coriander, cook for 1 minute, and then add the thyme, peppers, courgette, and garlic and cook for 5 minutes. Add the tomatoes, stock, and sherry. Season with black pepper, if needed, and bring to the boil. Return the chicken and chorizo, and cook in the oven for about 40 minutes until the chicken is tender when pierced with a fork. Serve with mashed sweet potatoes and peas.

Except for squid, seafood doesn't take kindly to slow cooking, so make the stew base first and add the fish at the last minute. For ease of preparation, you could always make this the day before.

Seafood stew

🔄 **SERVES** 4–6   ♡ **HEALTHY**

2 tbsp olive oil, plus extra for drizzling
1 onion, finely chopped
2 celery sticks, finely chopped
salt and freshly ground black pepper
1 tbsp dried oregano
1 fennel bulb, trimmed and roughly chopped
450g (1lb) cleaned squid, sliced into 1cm (½in) rings
350ml (12fl oz) dry white wine
2 lemons, zest peeled into strips using a
  vegetable peeler

1 tbsp tomato purée
400g can chopped tomatoes
600ml (1 pint) hot fish stock for the slow cooker
  (900ml/1½ pints for the traditional method)
1kg (2¼lb) mussels, scrubbed and debearded
  (discard any that do not close when tapped)
250g (9oz) raw shelled king prawns
350g (12oz) sea bass fillet (or other white fish such
  as haddock), skinned and cut into chunky pieces
few sprigs of flat-leaf parsley, finely chopped

in the slow cooker   🕐 **PREP** 20–30 MINS   **COOK** 15 MINS PRECOOKING; HIGH 3–4 HRS

1 Preheat the slow cooker, if required. Heat the oil in a large heavy-based pan over a medium heat, add the onion and celery, and cook for about 5 minutes until soft. Season with salt and pepper, then stir in the oregano and fennel and cook for a further 5 minutes.

2 Add the squid and cook over a low heat for a few minutes, stirring occasionally, then stir in the wine, and bring to the boil for 5 minutes. Stir in the strips of lemon zest and tomato purée, season well, and then add the canned tomatoes and stock. Transfer everything to the slow cooker, cover with the lid, and cook on high for 3–4 hours.

3 For the last 10 minutes of cooking, add the mussels, prawns, and sea bass, cover, and cook until the mussels have opened (discard any that do not open) and the fish is opaque and cooked through. Taste and season as needed. Ladle into deep, warmed bowls and serve with rice, couscous, or quinoa, a drizzle of olive oil, and a sprinkling of parsley.

traditional method   🕐 **PREP** 20–30 MINS   **COOK** 1½ HRS

1 Preheat the oven to 160°C (325°F/Gas 3). Heat the oil in a large flameproof casserole over a medium heat, add the onion and celery, and cook for about 5 minutes until soft. Season with salt and pepper, then stir in the oregano and fennel and cook for a further 5 minutes.

2 Add the squid and cook over a low heat for a few minutes, stirring occasionally, then stir in the wine, and bring to the boil for 5 minutes. Stir in the strips of lemon zest and tomato purée, season well, and then add the canned tomatoes and stock. Bring back to the boil, reduce to a simmer, cover, and put in the oven for 1 hour, topping up with hot stock if needed.

3 Add the mussels, prawns, and sea bass to the casserole, cover with the lid once more, and put back in the oven for 5 minutes or until the mussels have opened (discard any that do not open) and the fish is opaque and cooked through. Taste and season as needed. Ladle into deep, warmed bowls and serve with rice, couscous, or quinoa, a drizzle of olive oil, and a sprinkling of parsley.

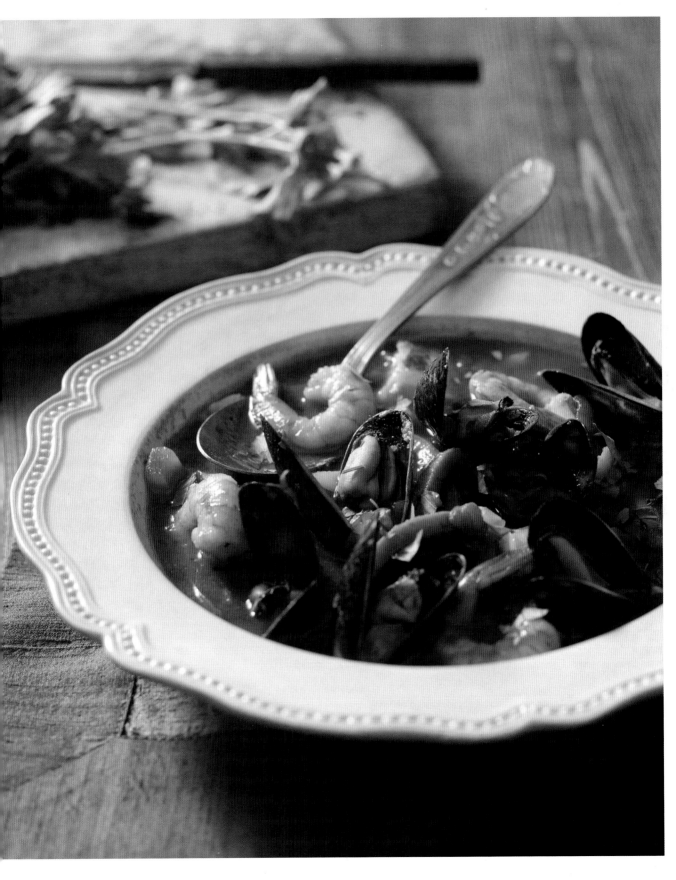

Duck legs are very succulent with lots of tasty meat on them. They can, however, be fatty so the addition of redcurrant jelly and raisins helps to balance this. Pine nuts give an added twist.

Duck legs with cabbage, pine nuts, and raisins

 SERVES 4–6

6 duck legs
2 red onions, roughly chopped
2 garlic cloves, finely chopped
few sprigs of thyme
1 bay leaf
1 tbsp redcurrant jelly

350ml (12fl oz) hot chicken stock for the slow cooker
 (600ml/1 pint for the traditional method)
salt and freshly ground black pepper
30g (1oz) raisins
30g (1oz) pine nuts, toasted
1 Savoy cabbage, cored and chopped into eighths

in the slow cooker   **PREP** 15 MINS   **COOK** 30 MINS PRECOOKING;
AUTO/LOW 6 HRS OR **HIGH** 3–4 HRS

1 Preheat the slow cooker, if required. Heat a large flameproof casserole over a medium heat, then add the duck legs and cook for 15–20 minutes, turning them as you go, until they begin to turn golden. Remove them from the casserole, set aside, and pour off any fat.

2 Add the onions, garlic, thyme, and bay leaf and cook for 5 minutes, then add the redcurrant jelly and cook for a few minutes more. Transfer everything to the slow cooker and add the duck legs, nestling them into the onion mixture, skin-side up. Pour over the stock, season with salt and pepper, cover with the lid, and cook on auto/low for 6 hours or on high for 3–4 hours.

3 Add the raisins, pine nuts, and cabbage to the casserole for the last 1 hour of cooking. Discard the bay leaf, taste, and adjust the seasoning. Serve with creamy mashed potatoes and some chilli jelly on the side.

traditional method   **PREP** 15 MINS   **COOK** 2½ HRS

1 Preheat the oven to 180°C (350°F/Gas 4). Heat a large flameproof casserole over a medium heat, then add the duck legs and cook for 15–20 minutes, turning them as you go, until they begin to turn golden. Remove them from the casserole, set aside, and pour off any fat.

2 Add the onions, garlic, thyme, and bay leaf and cook for 5 minutes, then add the redcurrant jelly and cook for a few minutes more. Return the duck legs to the casserole and nestle them into the onion mixture, skin-side up. Pour over the stock, bring to the boil, and then reduce to a simmer. Season with salt and pepper, cover with the lid, and put in the oven for 2 hours. Check occasionally that it's not drying out, topping up with a little hot water if needed.

3 Add the raisins, pine nuts, and cabbage to the casserole for the last 30 minutes of cooking. Discard the bay leaf, taste, and adjust the seasoning. Serve with creamy mashed potatoes and some chilli jelly on the side.

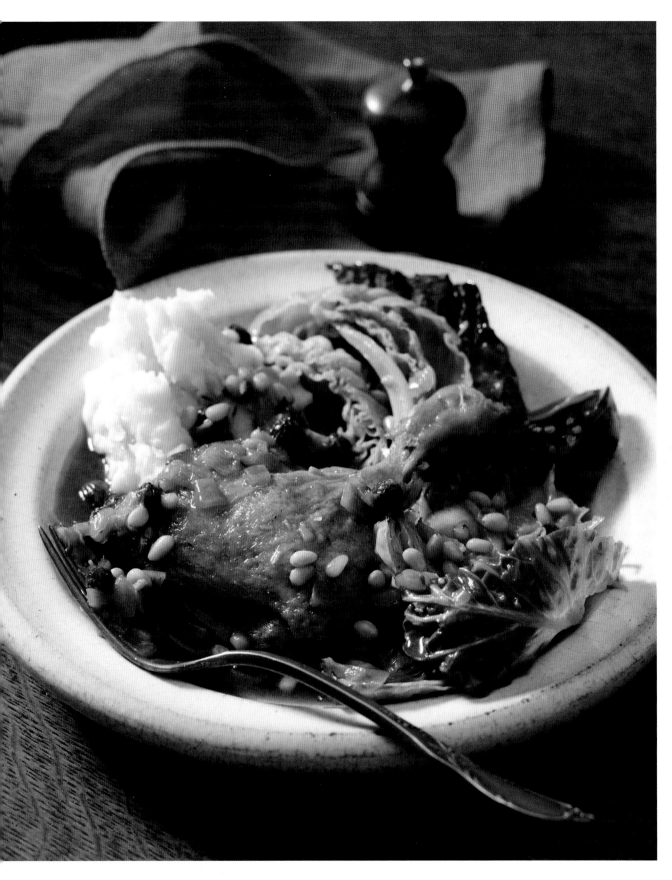

Rich and robust, oxtail makes a change to beef and braising it very slowly tenderizes it to the full. Prunes are always a tasty addition to a stew as their sweetness and texture complement the meat.

Braised oxtail with star anise

SERVES 4–6 **FREEZE** UP TO 3 MONTHS

2 oxtails, about 1.35kg (3lb) each, cut
  into bite-sized pieces
salt and freshly ground black pepper
2 tbsp olive oil
2 red onions, sliced
3 garlic clove, finely chopped
pinch of dried chilli flakes
350ml (12fl oz) red wine
4 star anise

handful of black peppercorns
1 bay leaf
8 soft prunes, stoned and chopped
600ml (1 pint) hot beef stock for the slow cooker
  (900ml/1½ pints for the traditional method)
4 clementines or 2 oranges, peeled and sliced
  into rings
small bunch of curly parsley leaves, finely chopped

in the slow cooker   PREP 20 MINS   COOK 15 MINS PRECOOKING; AUTO/LOW 8 HRS

1 Preheat the slow cooker, if required. Season the oxtail with salt and pepper. Heat half the oil in a large flameproof casserole over a medium heat, then add the meat in batches, and fry for 8–10 minutes until browned on all sides. Remove from the casserole and set aside.

2 Heat the remaining oil in the casserole over a medium heat, add the onions, and cook for 3–4 minutes to soften. Stir through the garlic and chilli flakes, then pour in the wine and let it simmer before adding it to the slow cooker together with the meat, star anise, peppercorns, bay leaf, prunes, and stock. Cover with the lid and cook on auto/low for 8 hours. Add the clementines for the last 30 minutes of cooking.

3 Shred the meat from the bone into the slow cooker, and discard the bone, bay leaf, and star anise. Serve on a bed of pasta, sprinkled with the parsley.

traditional method   PREP 20 MINS   COOK 3¼ HRS

1 Preheat the oven to 150°C (300°F/Gas 2). Season the oxtail with salt and pepper. Heat half the oil in a large flameproof casserole over a medium heat, then add the meat in batches, and fry for 8–10 minutes until browned on all sides. Remove with a slotted spoon and set aside.

2 Heat the remaining oil in the casserole over a medium heat, add the onions, and cook for 3–4 minutes to soften. Stir through the garlic and chilli flakes, then pour in the wine and let it simmer for about 5 minutes until slightly reduced. Return the meat to the casserole and add the star anise, peppercorns, bay leaf, and prunes, and pour over just enough stock to cover the meat.

3 Bring to the boil, then reduce to a simmer, add the remaining stock, cover, and put in the oven for about 3 hours. Check occasionally that it's not drying out, topping up with a little hot water if needed. Add the clementines or oranges for the last 30 minutes of cooking and leave the casserole uncovered to allow the liquid to thicken slightly. Stir it occasionally to keep the oxtail moist and coated with the gravy. When ready, the meat will fall away from the bone. Remove the bone and discard it together with the bay leaf and star anise. Serve on a bed of pasta, sprinkled with the parsley.

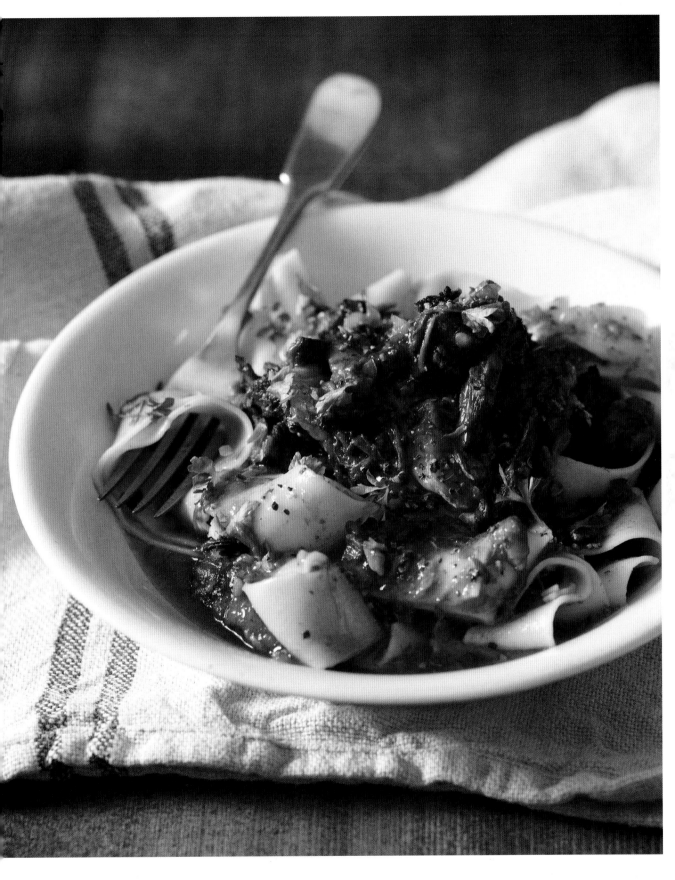

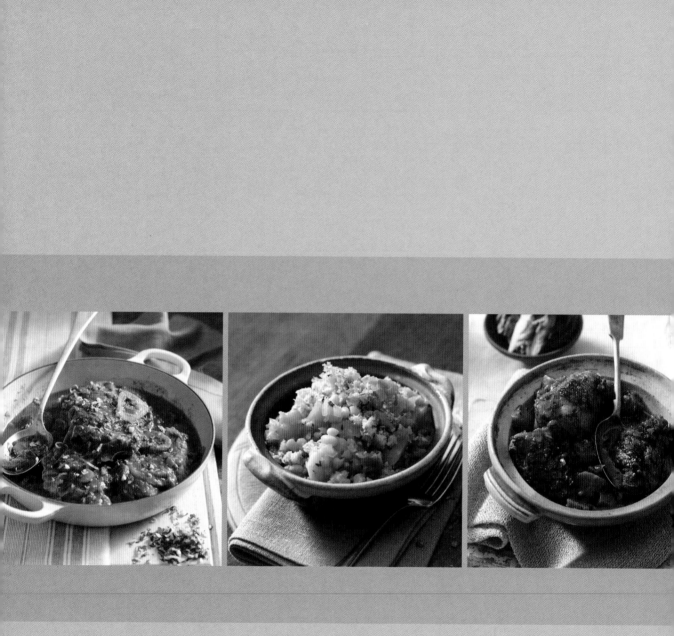

Casseroles & cassoulets

A robust dish that will hit the spot on cold days and fill you up. The lentils become soft and tender and, because they are cooked for so long, they are flavoured by the sausages.

Lentil and Toulouse sausage casserole

⊙ **SERVES** 4–6 ❄ **FREEZE** UP TO 1 MONTH

2 tbsp olive oil
8 Toulouse sausages, roughly chopped
1 onion, finely chopped
2 carrots, peeled and finely diced
freshly ground black pepper
3 garlic cloves, finely chopped
140g (5oz) chorizo, diced
3 sprigs of rosemary

few sprigs of thyme
200g (7oz) Puy lentils or brown lentils, rinsed and
   picked over for any stones
175ml (6fl oz) red wine
600ml (1 pint) hot chicken stock for the slow cooker
   (900ml/1½ pints for the traditional method)
1 red chilli, left whole
splash of extra virgin olive oil, to serve

in the slow cooker 🕒 **PREP** 15 MINS **COOK** 15 MINS PRECOOKING; **AUTO/LOW** 6–8 HRS

1 Preheat the slow cooker, if required. Heat half the oil in a large flameproof casserole over a high heat, add the Toulouse sausages, and cook for a few minutes until they begin to turn golden. Remove from the casserole and set aside.

2 Add the remaining oil, stir in the onion and carrot, and turn to coat. Season with pepper and leave to cook for a few minutes, stirring occasionally. Add the garlic, chorizo, and herbs, give it all a stir, then return the Toulouse sausages to the casserole and stir in the lentils. Add the wine, bring to the boil, and cook for a minute. Transfer everything to the slow cooker, add the chicken stock and chilli, cover with the lid, and cook on auto/low for 6–8 hours.

3 Taste and season, if necessary, remove the whole chilli, then ladle into warmed bowls and serve with a splash of extra virgin olive oil and some crusty bread.

traditional method 🕒 **PREP** 15 MINS **COOK** 1¾ HRS

1 Preheat the oven to 160°C (325°F/Gas 3). Heat half the oil in a large flameproof casserole over a high heat, add the Toulouse sausages, and cook for a few minutes until they begin to turn golden. Remove from the casserole and set aside.

2 Add the remaining oil, stir in the onion and carrot, and turn to coat. Season with pepper and leave to cook for a few minutes, stirring occasionally. Add the garlic, chorizo, and herbs, give it all a stir, then return the Toulouse sausages to the casserole and stir in the lentils. Add the wine, bring to the boil, and cook for a minute.

3 Pour in the stock, bring to the boil, then reduce to a simmer. Add the chilli, cover with the lid, and put in the oven for 1½ hours. Check occasionally that it's not drying out, topping up with a little hot water if needed. Taste and season, if necessary, remove the whole chilli, then ladle into warmed bowls and serve with a splash of extra virgin olive oil and some crusty bread.

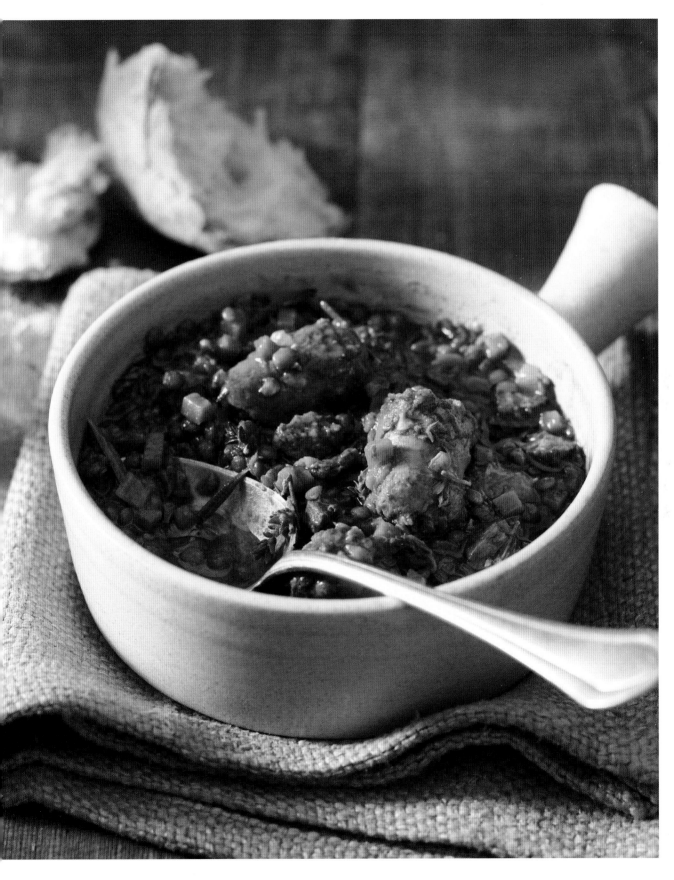

Look for ready-diced packs of game meat, which cut down on preparation time. Cider, carrot, and parsnip lend a sweetness to this dish and the fennel seeds add a welcome touch of aniseed.

Autumn game casserole

SERVES 4 **FREEZE** UP TO 3 MONTHS

2 tbsp olive oil
500g (1lb 2oz) mixed casserole game, such as
  pheasant, partridge, venison, rabbit, and
  pigeon, cut into bite-sized cubes
1 onion, chopped
1 carrot, peeled and chopped
1 parsnip, peeled and chopped
1 fennel bulb, diced, fronds reserved

2 tbsp plain flour
200ml (7fl oz) dry cider or apple juice
200ml (7fl oz) hot chicken stock, for both methods
250g (9oz) chestnut mushrooms, thickly sliced
½ tsp fennel seeds
salt and freshly ground black pepper
small handful of flat-leaf parsley, chopped (optional)

in the slow cooker PREP 20 MINS COOK 15 MINS PRECOOKING;
AUTO/LOW 6–8 HRS OR HIGH 2–3 HRS

1 Preheat the slow cooker, if required. Heat the oil in a large flameproof casserole over a medium-high heat and cook the game meat, stirring occasionally, for 3–4 minutes until lightly browned. Remove and set aside.

2 Lower the heat to medium, add the onion, carrot, parsnip, and fennel to the casserole and cook, stirring occasionally, for 4–5 minutes until lightly coloured. Sprinkle in the flour and gradually stir in the cider and stock. Add the mushrooms and fennel seeds, then bring to the boil. Transfer everything to the slow cooker, including the game meat, season well, and cover with the lid. Cook on auto/low for 6–8 hours or on high for 2–3 hours. Sprinkle the finished dish with the reserved fennel fronds or chopped parsley and serve hot with some creamy mashed potatoes.

traditional method PREP 20 MINS COOK 1½ HRS

1 Preheat the oven to 160°C (325°C/Gas 3). Heat the oil in a large flameproof casserole over a medium-high heat and cook the game meat, stirring occasionally, for 3–4 minutes until lightly browned. Remove and set aside.

2 Lower the heat to medium, add the onion, carrot, parsnip, and fennel to the casserole and cook, stirring occasionally, for 4–5 minutes until lightly coloured. Sprinkle in the flour and gradually stir in the cider and stock. Add the mushrooms and fennel seeds, then return the meat, season well, and bring to the boil. Cover tightly with the lid and put in the oven for about 1¼ hours, or until the meat and vegetables are tender. Sprinkle the finished dish with the reserved fennel fronds or chopped parsley and serve hot with some creamy mashed potatoes.

Try using a Normandy cider for this dish, for an authentic flavour. Crème fraîche can be used in place of the cream. Stir through a handful of walnuts at the end to add flavour.

Pork Normandy

SERVES 4–6

2 tbsp olive oil
knob of butter
900g (2lb) lean pork, cut into bite-sized pieces
2 onions, finely chopped
2 tbsp Dijon mustard
4 garlic cloves, finely chopped
4 celery sticks, finely chopped
3 carrots, peeled and finely chopped

1 tbsp chopped rosemary leaves
2 Bramley apples, peeled, cored, and roughly chopped
200ml (7fl oz) dry cider
200ml (7fl oz) hot light chicken stock, for both methods
200ml (7fl oz) double cream
1 tsp black peppercorns

in the slow cooker   **PREP** 30 MINS   **COOK** 25 MINS PRECOOKING; AUTO/LOW 6–8 HRS OR HIGH 3–4 HRS

1 Preheat the slow cooker, if required. Heat the oil and butter in a large flameproof casserole over a medium heat, add the pork (in batches, if necessary), and cook for about 10 minutes, stirring occasionally, until golden brown on all sides. Remove and set aside.

2 Reduce the heat to low, add the onions, and cook for about 5 minutes until soft. Stir in the mustard, garlic, celery, carrots, and rosemary, and cook, stirring often, for about 10 minutes until tender. Add the apples and cook for a further 5 minutes.

3 Pour in the cider, increase the heat, and boil for a couple of minutes while the alcohol evaporates. Transfer everything to the slow cooker, including the pork, and pour over the stock. Cover with the lid and cook on auto/low for 6–8 hours or on high for 3–4 hours. Add the cream and peppercorns for the last 20 minutes of cooking. Serve with fluffy rice or creamy mashed potatoes.

traditional method   **PREP** 30 MINS   **COOK** 1½ HRS

1 Preheat the oven to 180°C (350°F/Gas 4). Heat the oil and butter in a large flameproof casserole over a medium heat, add the pork (in batches, if necessary), and cook for about 10 minutes, stirring occasionally, until golden brown on all sides. Remove and set aside.

2 Reduce the heat to low, add the onions, and cook for about 5 minutes until soft. Stir in the mustard, garlic, celery, carrots, and rosemary, and cook, stirring often, for about 10 minutes until tender. Add the apples and cook for a further 5 minutes.

3 Pour in the cider, increase the heat, and boil for a couple of minutes while the alcohol evaporates. Return the pork to the casserole and pour in the stock and cream. Stir in the peppercorns, bring to the boil, cover with the lid, and put in the oven for 1 hour, or until the sauce has reduced and the pork is tender. Serve with fluffy rice or creamy mashed potatoes.

This Italian classic is served with a zesty gremolata, and it would be delicious with a saffron and Parmesan risotto. Ask your butcher for a hindleg of veal as they are meatier than the front legs.

Osso bucco

SERVES 4–6

30g (1oz) plain flour
salt and freshly ground black pepper
4–6 pieces of veal shin on the bone (about 1.8kg/4lb)
2 tbsp vegetable oil
30g (1oz) butter
1 carrot, peeled and thinly sliced
2 onions, finely chopped
250ml (9fl oz) white wine
400g can Italian plum tomatoes, drained and
  coarsely chopped

1 garlic clove, finely chopped
finely grated zest of 1 orange
120ml (4fl oz) hot chicken or veal stock for
  both methods

FOR THE GREMOLATA
small bunch of flat-leaf parsley, leaves
  finely chopped
finely grated zest of 1 lemon
1 garlic clove, finely chopped

in the slow cooker   PREP 15 MINS   COOK 15 MINS PRECOOKING;
AUTO/LOW 6–8 HRS OR HIGH 4 HRS

1 Preheat the slow cooker, if required. Put the flour on a large plate, season with salt and pepper, and stir to combine. Lightly coat the veal pieces with the seasoned flour. Heat the oil and butter in a large flameproof casserole over a medium heat, add the veal pieces (in batches and with extra oil, if necessary), and brown thoroughly on all sides. Transfer to a plate with a slotted spoon and set aside.

2 Add the carrot and onions and cook, stirring occasionally, until soft. Add the wine and boil until reduced by half. Stir in the tomatoes, garlic, and orange zest, and add seasoning. Transfer everything to the slow cooker, then lay the veal on top, and pour over the stock. Cover with the lid and cook for 6–8 hours on auto/low or on high for 4 hours.

3 For the gremolata, mix the parsley, lemon, and garlic in a small bowl. Put the veal on warmed plates, spoon the sauce on top and sprinkle with the gremolata.

traditional method   PREP 30–35 MINS   COOK 1¾–2¼ HRS

1 Preheat the oven to 180°C (350°F/Gas 4). Put the flour on a large plate, season with salt and pepper, and stir to combine. Lightly coat the veal pieces with the seasoned flour. Heat the oil and butter in a large flameproof casserole over a medium heat, add the veal pieces (in batches and with extra oil, if necessary), and brown thoroughly on all sides. Transfer to a plate with a slotted spoon and set aside.

2 Add the carrot and onions and cook, stirring occasionally, until soft. Add the wine and boil until reduced by half. Stir in the tomatoes, garlic, and orange zest, and add seasoning. Transfer everything to the slow cooker, then lay the veal on top, and pour over the stock. Cover with the lid and put in the oven for 1½–2 hours until very tender. Check occasionally that it's not drying out, topping up with a little hot water if needed.

3 For the gremolata, mix the parsley, lemon, and garlic in a small bowl. Put the veal on warmed plates, spoon the sauce on top and sprinkle with the gremolata.

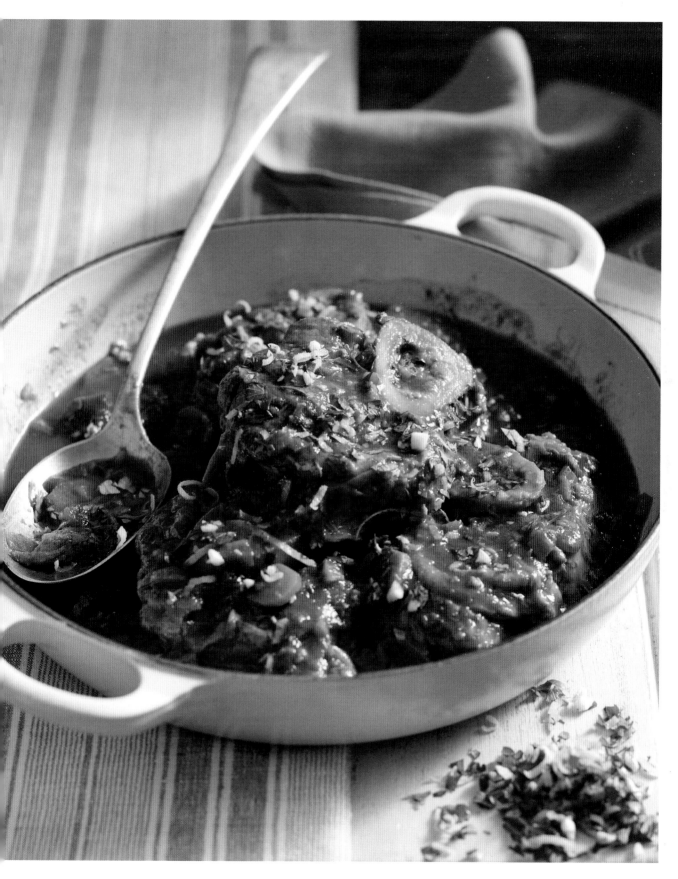

In this classic French casserole, long, slow braising ensures the meat becomes tender, cooked as it is in red wine. Traditionally, the French use red Burgundy wine, but it's not obligatory.

Boeuf bourguignon

SERVES 4 **FREEZE** UP TO 3 MONTHS

175g (6oz) streaky bacon rashers, chopped
1–2 tbsp olive oil
900g (2lb) braising steak, cut into 4cm (1½in) cubes
12 small shallots, peeled and left whole
1 tbsp plain flour
300ml (10fl oz) red wine
200ml (7fl oz) hot beef stock for the slow cooker
 (300ml/10fl oz for the traditional method)

115g (4oz) button mushrooms
1 bay leaf
1 tsp dried herbes de Provence
salt and freshly ground black pepper
4 tbsp chopped flat-leaf parsley

in the slow cooker **PREP** 20 MINS **COOK** 20 MINS PRECOOKING; **AUTO/LOW** 6–8 HRS

1 Preheat the slow cooker, if required. Fry the bacon in a large flameproof casserole over a medium heat until lightly browned. Drain on kitchen paper, then set aside and keep warm. Depending on how much fat is left from the bacon, add a little oil to the casserole, if necessary, so you have 2–3 tbsp, and increase the heat to high. Fry the beef (in batches, if necessary) for 8–10 minutes until browned all over. Remove, set aside, and keep warm. Reduce the heat to medium and fry the shallots for 6–8 minutes and then remove these too, and set aside with the meat.

2 Stir the flour into the remaining fat in the casserole. If the casserole is quite dry, mix the flour with a little of the wine or stock. Pour the remaining wine and stock into the casserole and bring to the boil, stirring until smooth. Add the mushrooms, bay leaf, and dried herbs. Add seasoning and then transfer everything to the slow cooker, including the bacon, beef, and shallots. Cover with the lid and cook on auto/low for 6–8 hours. Sprinkle with the chopped parsley, remove the bay leaf, and serve with mashed potatoes, baby carrots, and a green vegetable such as broccoli or French beans.

traditional method **PREP** 25 MINS **COOK** 2½ HRS

1 Preheat the oven to 160°C (325°F/Gas 3). Fry the bacon in a large flameproof casserole over a medium heat until lightly browned. Drain on kitchen paper, then set aside and keep warm. Depending on how much fat is left from the bacon, add a little oil to the casserole, if necessary, so you have 2–3 tbsp, and increase the heat to high. Fry the beef (in batches, if necessary) for 8–10 minutes until browned all over. Remove, set aside, and keep warm. Reduce the heat to medium and fry the shallots for 6–8 minutes and then remove these too, and set aside with the meat.

2 Stir the flour into the remaining fat in the casserole. If the casserole is quite dry, mix the flour with a little of the wine or stock. Pour the remaining wine and stock into the casserole and bring to the boil, stirring until smooth. Add the mushrooms, bay leaf, and dried herbs. Add seasoning and return the meat and shallots to the casserole. Cover and cook in the oven for 2 hours, or until the meat is very tender. Check occasionally that it's not drying out, topping up with a little hot water if needed.

3 Sprinkle with the chopped parsley, remove the bay leaf, and serve with mashed potatoes, baby carrots, and a green vegetable such as broccoli or French beans.

The flavour varies with the wine used: a Rhône wine gives a rich sauce; a Loire wine, a fruitier dish. Start the recipe a day ahead to allow time for marinating. Serve with new potatoes.

Coq au vin

SERVES 4–6

1 onion, thinly sliced
1 celery stick, thinly sliced
1 carrot, peeled and thinly sliced
2 garlic cloves, 1 peeled and left whole, 1 finely chopped
6 black peppercorns
375ml (13fl oz) red wine
2kg (4½lb) chicken, jointed into 8 pieces
2 tbsp olive oil
1 tbsp vegetable oil

15g (½oz) butter
125g (4½oz) piece of bacon, diced
18–20 baby onions, peeled
3 tbsp flour
500ml (16fl oz) hot chicken stock, for both methods
2 shallots, finely chopped
1 bouquet garni
salt and freshly ground black pepper
250g (9oz) mushrooms, quartered

in the slow cooker   **PREP** 30 MINS, PLUS MARINATING   **COOK** 20 MINS PRECOOKING; **AUTO/LOW** 6–8 HRS OR **HIGH** 3–4 HRS

1 For the marinade, put the onion, celery, carrot, whole garlic clove, and peppercorns in a pan. Pour in the wine and bring to the boil. Simmer for about 5 minutes, then cool and pour into a large bowl. Add the chicken and olive oil, cover, and refrigerate for 12–18 hours, turning the chicken occasionally.

2 Preheat the slow cooker, if required. Remove the chicken from the marinade and dry on kitchen paper. Strain the marinade and reserve the liquid and vegetables. Heat the vegetable oil and butter in a flameproof casserole until foaming. Add the bacon, brown it, remove, and set aside. Add the chicken and cook for 10–15 minutes until brown. Remove and set aside. Discard all but 2 tbsp of the fat. Reduce the heat to medium and cook the baby onions for 3–4 minutes until soft. Add the reserved vegetables and cook over a very low heat for 5 minutes until soft. Add the flour and cook for 2 minutes until lightly browned. Stir in the reserved marinade, stock, chopped garlic, shallots, bouquet garni, and seasoning. Bring to the boil, then transfer to the slow cooker, adding the bacon and chicken. Cover with the lid and cook on auto/low for 6–8 hours or on high for 3–4 hours. Add the mushrooms with 15 minutes remaining.

traditional method   **PREP** 30 MINS, PLUS MARINATING   **COOK** 1½–1¾ HRS

1 For the marinade, put the onion, celery, carrot, whole garlic clove, and peppercorns in a pan. Pour in the wine and bring to the boil. Simmer for about 5 minutes, then cool and pour into a large bowl. Add the chicken and olive oil, cover, and refrigerate for 12–18 hours, turning the chicken occasionally.

2 Remove the chicken from the marinade and dry on kitchen paper. Strain the marinade and reserve the liquid and vegetables. Heat the vegetable oil and butter in a flameproof casserole until foaming. Add the bacon, brown it, remove, and set aside. Add the chicken and cook for 10–15 minutes until brown. Remove and set aside. Discard all but 2 tbsp of the fat. Reduce the heat to medium and cook the baby onions for 3–4 minutes until soft. Add the reserved vegetables and cook over a low heat for 5 minutes until soft. Add the flour and cook for 2 minutes until lightly browned. Stir in the reserved marinade, stock, chopped garlic, shallots, bouquet garni, and seasoning. Bring to the boil. Return the chicken, cover, and simmer over a low heat for 45–60 minutes until tender. Add the mushrooms with 15 minutes remaining.

This popular Mediterranean dish makes an easy vegetarian supper. Make ahead so the flavours become well acquainted, then reheat to serve. Any leftovers are just as good served cold.

Ratatouille

⊙ **SERVES** 4 ❄ **FREEZE** UP TO 3 MONTHS

4 tbsp olive oil
1 small aubergine, about 225g (8oz), chopped
   into 2.5cm (1in) cubes
1 courgette, trimmed and sliced
1 onion, chopped
1 garlic clove, chopped

1 red pepper, deseeded and chopped into 2.5cm
   (1in) pieces
150ml (5fl oz) hot vegetable stock, for both methods
400g can chopped tomatoes
2 tsp chopped oregano, plus 2–3 sprigs to serve
salt and freshly ground black pepper

in the slow cooker 🕐 **PREP** 15 MINS **COOK** 30 MINS PRECOOKING;
                                                                    AUTO/LOW 4–5 HRS OR **HIGH** 2–3 HRS

1 Preheat the slow cooker, if required. Heat half the oil in a large heavy-based pan over a medium heat, add the aubergine, and cook for about 10 minutes until beginning to colour. Remove and set aside. Add the courgette, with more oil if necessary, and cook for 5–8 minutes until golden. Remove and set aside. Now add the onion together with any remaining oil, and cook for 4–5 minutes until soft. Stir in the garlic and peppers and cook for about 5 minutes to soften.

2 Pour in the stock and tomatoes with their juice, stir in the chopped oregano, and bring to the boil. Transfer to the slow cooker, cover with the lid, and cook on auto/low for 4–5 hours or on high for 2–3 hours. Stir through the aubergine and courgette for the last 30 minutes of cooking.

3 Taste and add seasoning, if needed. Spoon the ratatouille into a warmed serving bowl and top with the oregano sprigs. Serve with rice, bulgur wheat, or couscous, and sprinkle some grated cheese over the ratatouille, if you wish.

traditional method 🕐 **PREP** 15 MINS **COOK** 1¼ HRS

1 Heat half the oil in a large heavy-based pan over a medium heat, add the aubergine, and cook for about 10 minutes until beginning to colour. Remove and set aside. Add the courgette, with more oil if necessary, and cook for 5–8 minutes until golden. Also remove and set aside. Now add the onion together with any remaining oil, and cook for 4–5 minutes until soft. Stir in the garlic and peppers and cook for about 5 minutes to soften.

2 Pour in the stock and tomatoes with their juice, stir in the chopped oregano, and bring to the boil. Reduce the heat to low and partially cover with the lid. Cook, stirring occasionally, for about 40 minutes, topping up with a little hot water if needed. Stir through the aubergine and courgette, and simmer for 10 minutes more.

3 Taste and add seasoning, if needed. Spoon the ratatouille into a warmed serving bowl and top with the oregano sprigs. Serve with rice, bulgur wheat, or couscous, and sprinkle some grated cheese over the ratatouille, if you wish.

This is a hearty bean and meat dish from southwest France. Use dried beans if you prefer, but they will need overnight soaking and boiling for 10 minutes before adding to the casserole.

Cassoulet de Toulouse

SERVES 4   **FREEZE** UP TO 3 MONTHS

1 tbsp olive oil
2 duck legs
4 Toulouse sausages
150g (5½oz) piece of pancetta or a whole chorizo
   sausage, chopped into small pieces
1 onion, peeled and finely chopped
1 carrot, peeled and chopped
4 garlic cloves, crushed
2 x 400g cans haricot beans, drained and rinsed

1 sprig of thyme, plus ½ tbsp chopped leaves
1 bay leaf
salt and freshly ground black pepper
2 tbsp tomato purée
400g can chopped tomatoes
150ml (5fl oz) white wine
½ day-old baguette, crusts removed and torn
   into pieces
1 tbsp chopped parsley

in the slow cooker   **PREP** 30 MINS   **COOK** 50 MINS PRECOOKING; AUTO/LOW 6–8 HRS

1 Preheat the slow cooker, if required. Heat the oil in a large flameproof casserole over a medium-high heat and add the duck legs, skin-side down. Cook each side for 3–6 minutes until golden. Remove and reserve the duck fat. Add the sausages, cook for 7–8 minutes until browned, then remove and set aside. Cook the pancetta for 5 minutes and also remove and set aside. Add the onions and carrot, cook over a medium heat for 10 minutes until soft, then cook most of the garlic for 1 minute. Layer the ingredients in the slow cooker, beginning with half the beans, then the onion, carrot, sausages, pancetta, and duck legs, followed by the remaining beans, and adding the bay leaf and thyme as you go. Season with salt and pepper. Mix 400ml (14fl oz) of hot water with the tomato purée, tomatoes, and wine, then add to the slow cooker. Cover with the lid and cook on auto/low for 6–8 hours.

2 Put the baguette in a food processor with the remaining garlic. Process into coarse crumbs. Heat 2 tbsp of the duck fat in a heavy-based pan over a medium heat and fry the crumbs for 7–8 minutes until golden. Drain on kitchen paper and stir in the parsley. Sprinkle over the cassoulet and serve.

traditional method   **PREP** 30 MINS   **COOK** 3¾ HRS

1 Preheat the oven to 140°C (275°F/Gas 1). Heat the oil in a large flameproof casserole over a medium-high heat and add the duck legs, skin-side down. Cook each side for 3–6 minutes until golden. Remove and reserve the duck fat. Add the sausages, cook for 7–8 minutes until browned, then remove and set aside. Cook the pancetta for 5 minutes and also remove and set aside. Add the onions and carrot, cook over a medium heat for 10 minutes until soft, then cook most of the garlic for 1 minute. Layer the ingredients in the casserole, beginning with half the beans, then onions, carrot, sausages, pancetta, and duck legs, followed by the remaining beans, and adding the bay leaf and thyme as you go. Season with salt and pepper. Mix 900ml (1½ pints) hot water with the tomato purée, tomatoes, and wine, then add to the casserole. Cover and cook in the oven for 3 hours, adding extra water if required.

2 Put the baguette in a food processor with the remaining garlic. Process into coarse crumbs. Heat 2 tbsp of the duck fat in a heavy-based pan over a medium heat and fry the crumbs for 7–8 minutes until golden. Drain on kitchen paper and stir in the parsley. Sprinkle over the cassoulet and serve.

Dumplings are the perfect addition to a casserole or stew as they make the dish a complete meal. For variety, add other herbs, such as thyme or tarragon, to the parsley in the mixture.

Vegetable casserole with dumplings

SERVES 4–6 ❄ **FREEZE** UP TO 1 MONTH

1 tbsp olive oil
1 onion, roughly chopped
salt and freshly ground black pepper
3 garlic cloves, finely chopped
pinch of dried chilli flakes
2 leeks, trimmed and thickly sliced
3 carrots, peeled and roughly chopped
2 celery sticks, roughly chopped

1 tbsp plain flour
600ml (1 pint) hot vegetable stock for the slow cooker (900ml/1½ pints for the traditional method)
400g can haricot beans, drained and rinsed
few sprigs of rosemary
225g (8oz) self-raising flour
115g (4oz) vegetable suet
2 tbsp finely chopped flat-leaf parsley

in the slow cooker 🕒 PREP 25 MINS   COOK 20 MINS PRECOOKING; AUTO/LOW 6–8 HRS OR HIGH 4 HRS

1 Preheat the slow cooker, if required. Heat the oil in a large heavy-based pan over a medium heat, add the onion, and cook for 3–4 minutes until soft. Season with salt and pepper, then stir through the garlic and chilli flakes. Add the leeks, carrots, and celery and continue cooking for a further 10 minutes, stirring occasionally, until softened. Stir in the plain flour, then gradually stir in the stock. Add the haricot beans and rosemary, and transfer everything to the slow cooker. Cover with the lid and cook on auto/low for 6–8 hours or on high for 4 hours.

2 About 45 minutes before the end of the cooking time, prepare the dumplings. Mix together the self-raising flour, suet, and parsley and season well. Add about 120ml (4fl oz) cold water to form a soft, slightly sticky dough, trickling in more water if it seems too dry. Form into 12 balls and drop them into the stew for the last 30 minutes of cooking. Push them down a little so they are just immersed and cover with the lid. Remove the rosemary, ladle the casserole into warmed bowls, and serve with crusty bread.

traditional method 🕒 PREP 25 MINS   COOK 1¼ HRS

1 Preheat the oven to 160°C (325°F/Gas 3). Heat the oil in a large flameproof casserole over a medium heat, add the onion, and cook for 3–4 minutes until soft. Season with salt and pepper, then stir through the garlic and chilli flakes. Add the leek, carrots, and celery and continue cooking for a further 10 minutes, stirring occasionally, until softened. Stir in the plain flour, then gradually stir in the stock. Add the haricot beans and rosemary. Bring to the boil, then reduce to a simmer, cover, and put in the oven for 1 hour, checking on the liquid level as it cooks and topping up with hot stock if needed.

2 While this is cooking, prepare the dumplings. Mix together the self-raising flour, suet, and parsley and season well. Add about 120ml (4fl oz) cold water to form a soft, slightly sticky dough, trickling in more water if it seems too dry. Form into 12 balls and drop them into the stew for the last 30 minutes of cooking. Push them down a little so they are just immersed and cover with the lid. Remove the lid for the final 10 minutes or until the dumplings are browned. Remove the rosemary, ladle the casserole into warmed bowls, and serve with crusty bread.

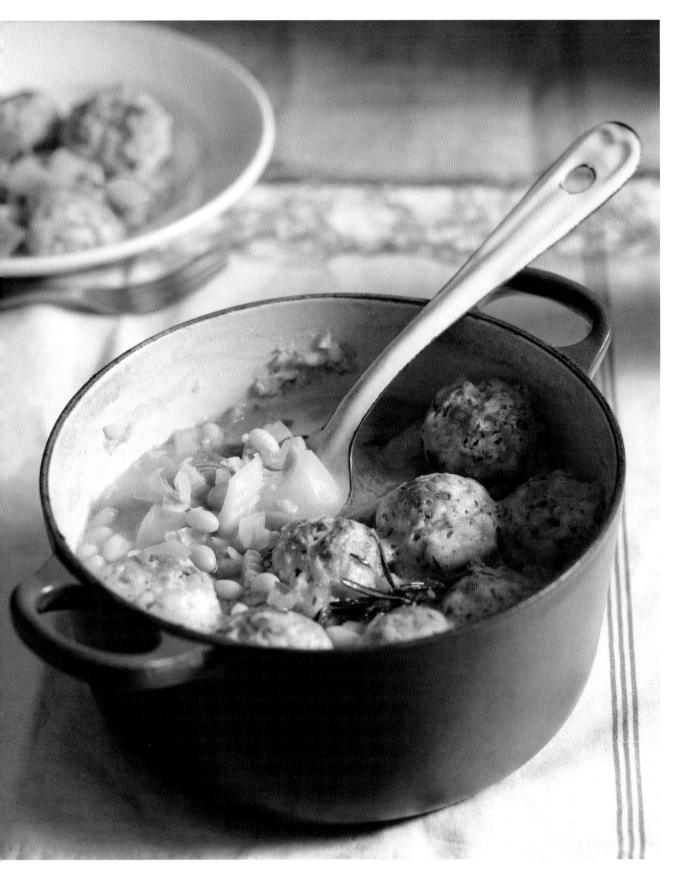

This is a lighter, vegetarian version of the traditional meaty cassoulet, featuring creamy haricot beans and a crispy, herby breadcrumb and Parmesan cheese topping.

Pumpkin and parsnip cassoulet

SERVES 4–6   **FREEZE** UP TO 3 MONTHS   **HEALTHY**

2 tbsp olive oil
1 onion, finely chopped
salt and freshly ground black pepper
3 garlic cloves, finely chopped
1 tsp ground cloves
2 carrots, peeled and finely chopped
2 celery sticks, finely chopped
1 bay leaf
450g (1lb) pumpkin (prepared weight), chopped
   into bite-sized pieces
450g (1lb) small parsnips, sliced into rounds

250ml (9fl oz) white wine
few sprigs of thyme
4 tomatoes, chopped, or use a 400g can tomatoes
400g can haricot beans, rinsed and drained
300ml (10fl oz) hot vegetable stock for the slow
   cooker (900ml/1½ pints for the traditional method)

FOR THE TOPPING
125g (4½oz) breadcrumbs, lightly toasted
30g (1oz) Parmesan cheese, grated
1 tbsp chopped flat-leaf parsley

in the slow cooker   PREP 15 MINS   COOK 20 MINS PRECOOKING;
AUTO/LOW 8 HRS OR HIGH 4 HRS

1 Preheat the slow cooker, if required. Heat the oil in a large heavy-based pan over a medium heat, add the onion, and cook for 3–4 minutes until soft. Season with salt and pepper, add the garlic, cloves, carrots, celery, and bay leaf, and cook, stirring occasionally, on a very low heat for 8–10 minutes until it is all soft. Stir through the pumpkin and parsnip and cook for a few minutes more, then pour in the wine. Increase the heat, stir, and let it bubble for a minute or two. Then add the thyme, tomatoes, and beans.

2 Transfer everything to the slow cooker, pour over the stock, season, and stir. Cover with the lid and cook on auto/low for 8 hours or on high for 4 hours. An hour before the end of the cooking time, mix the topping ingredients together in a bowl, sprinkle over, and replace the lid. Ladle into warmed bowls and serve with crusty bread.

traditional method   PREP 15 MINS   COOK 1¾ HRS

1 Preheat the oven to 180°C (350°F/Gas 4). Heat the oil in a large flameproof casserole over a medium heat, add the onion, and cook for 3–4 minutes until soft. Season with salt and pepper, add the garlic, cloves, carrots, celery, and bay leaf, and cook, stirring occasionally, on a very low heat for 8–10 minutes until it is all soft. Stir through the pumpkin and parsnip and cook for a few minutes more, then pour in the wine. Increase the heat, stir, and let it bubble for a minute or two. Then add the thyme, tomatoes, beans, and stock, and bring to the boil. Reduce to a simmer, season, cover with the lid, and put in the oven for 40 minutes.

2 Mix together the topping ingredients in a bowl, sprinkle it over the cassoulet and put back in the oven for 30 minutes. Then remove the lid and cook for about 10 minutes until the topping is golden. Ladle into warmed bowls and serve with crusty bread.

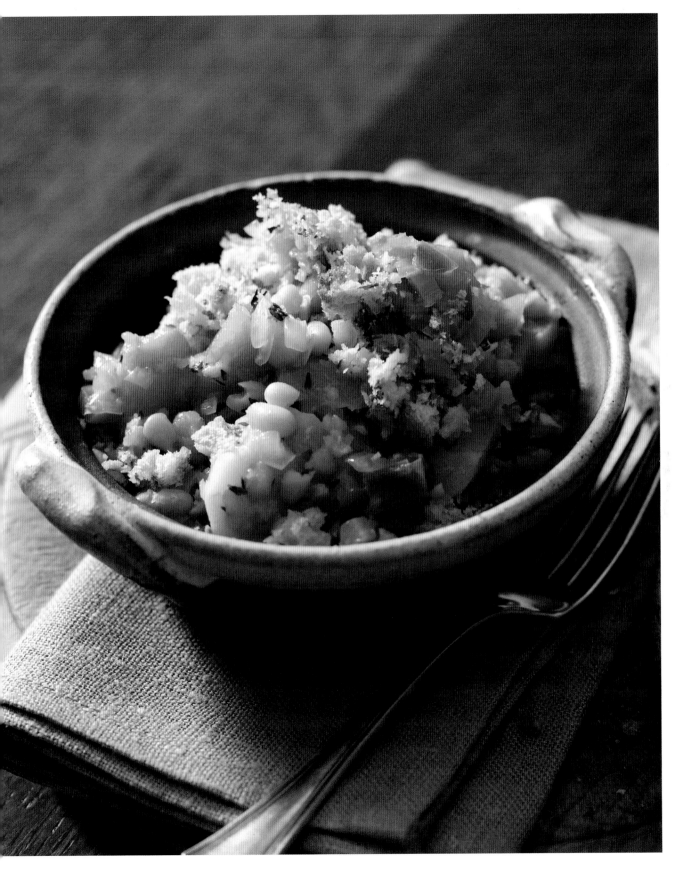

Dried fruit works well with a fatty meat such as pork belly – it creates a delicious, sweet sauce that cuts through the richness. The earthiness of celeriac is a great addition.

Belly pork and prunes

SERVES 4–6

1 tbsp olive oil
1.1kg (2½lb) pork belly, cut into bite-sized pieces
salt and freshly ground black pepper
1 onion, finely sliced
3 garlic cloves, finely chopped
1 tbsp sherry vinegar
120ml (4fl oz) white wine

600ml (1 pint) hot vegetable stock for the slow cooker (900ml/1½ pints for the traditional method)
140g (5oz) soft prunes, finely chopped
6 sage leaves, finely shredded
600g (1lb 5oz) celeriac, peeled and chopped into bite-sized pieces

in the slow cooker PREP 15 MINS COOK 30 MINS PRECOOKING; AUTO/LOW 8 HRS

1 Preheat the slow cooker, if required. Heat half the oil in a large flameproof casserole over a high heat and season the pork belly with salt and pepper. Add the pork (in batches, if necessary), skin-side down, and cook until it turns golden and begins to crisp a little. Remove and sit the pork on kitchen paper to drain.

2 Heat the remaining oil in the casserole over a medium heat, add the onion, and cook for 3–4 minutes until soft. Then stir in the garlic and cook for a minute more. Increase the heat and add the sherry vinegar, letting it simmer for 2–3 minutes. Pour in the wine and continue to boil for a few more minutes until the alcohol evaporates.

3 Transfer everything to the slow cooker, including the pork. Pour over the stock and stir in the prunes, sage, and celeriac. Cover with the lid and cook on auto/low for 8 hours. Taste and season more if needed, and serve with creamy mashed potatoes.

traditional method PREP 15 MINS COOK 3–3½ HRS

1 Preheat the oven to 160°C (325°F/Gas 3). Heat half the oil in a large flameproof casserole over a high heat and season the pork belly with salt and pepper. Add the pork (in batches, if necessary), skin-side down, and cook until it turns golden and begins to crisp a little. Remove and sit the pork on kitchen paper to drain.

2 Heat the remaining oil in the casserole over a medium heat, add the onion, and cook for 3–4 minutes until soft. Then stir in the garlic and cook for a minute more. Increase the heat and add the sherry vinegar, letting it simmer for 2–3 minutes. Pour in the wine and continue to boil for a few more minutes until the alcohol evaporates.

3 Add the stock and stir to scrape up the bits from the bottom of the casserole. Return the pork to the casserole and stir in the prunes, sage, and celeriac. Bring back to the boil, cover, and put in the oven for 2½–3 hours. Check occasionally that it's not drying out, topping up with a little hot water if needed. Taste and season more if needed, and serve with creamy mashed potatoes.

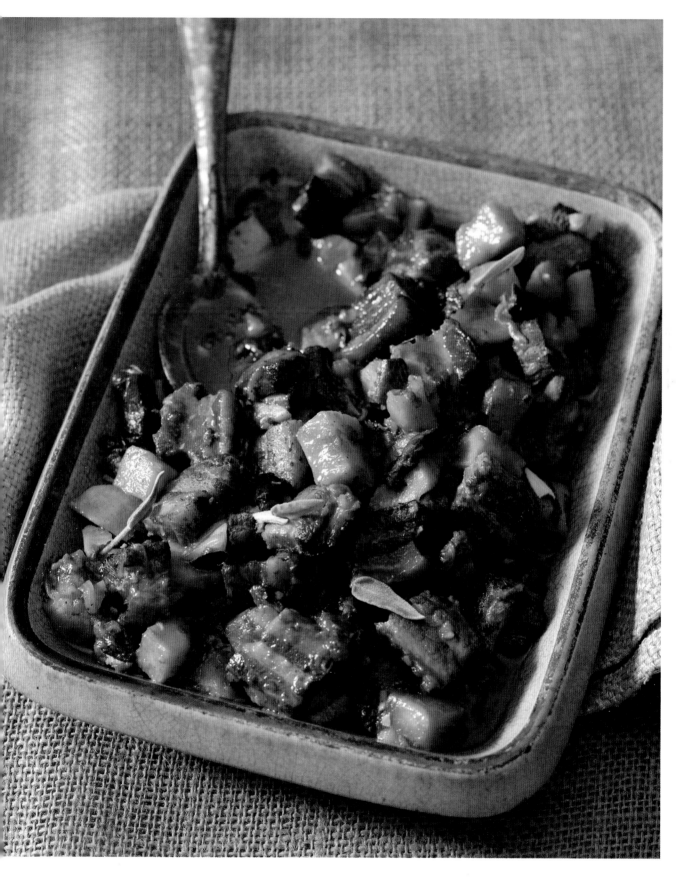

There are numerous versions of the "daube", but all are cooked in red wine. Choose a robust wine that you would happily drink. Throw in a cinnamon stick, if you wish, for a touch of warm spice.

Provençal lamb daube with olives

⊚ **SERVES** 4–6   ❄ **FREEZE** UP TO 3 MONTHS

1 orange, zest peeled in wide strips
2 garlic cloves, finely chopped
500ml (16fl oz) red wine
2 bay leaves
3–4 sprigs each of rosemary, thyme, and parsley
10 peppercorns
900g (2lb) boned lamb shoulder, cut into large cubes
2 tbsp olive oil
salt and freshly ground black pepper

300g (10oz) piece of smoked streaky bacon, cut into 5mm (¼in) lardons
400g can chopped tomatoes
2 onions, sliced
2 carrots, peeled and sliced
175g (6oz) mushrooms, trimmed and sliced
140g (5oz) stoned green olives
200ml (7fl oz) hot beef stock for the slow cooker (250ml/9fl oz for the traditional method)

in the slow cooker   ⏱ **PREP** 15 MINS, PLUS MARINATING   **COOK** 10 MINS PRECOOKING; AUTO/LOW 6–8 HRS

1 To make the marinade, combine the orange zest, garlic, wine, bay leaves, herbs, and peppercorns in a bowl. Add the lamb and mix well. Pour the oil on top and add seasoning. Cover and refrigerate, turning occasionally, and leave to marinate for 2 hours or up to 12 hours if time permits.

2 Preheat the slow cooker, if required. Put the bacon in a large heavy-based pan of water, bring to the boil, and blanch for 5 minutes. Drain and rinse with cold water. Remove the lamb from the marinade and dry on kitchen paper. Strain the marinade, reserving the liquid, bay leaf, and zest.

3 Put the bacon on the bottom of the slow cooker and cover with the lamb. Layer the tomatoes and onions on top, then the carrots, mushrooms, and olives. Pour in the strained marinade and stock, season with pepper, and add the bay leaf and zest. Cover with the lid and cook on auto/low for 6–8 hours. Remove the bay leaf and zest, taste, and season if needed. Serve with mashed potatoes.

traditional method   ⏱ **PREP** 45–50 MINS, PLUS MARINATING   **COOK** 3¾–4¼ HRS

1 To make the marinade, combine the orange zest, garlic, wine, bay leaves, herbs, and peppercorns in a bowl. Add the lamb and mix well. Pour the oil on top and add seasoning. Cover and refrigerate, turning occasionally, and leave to marinate for 2 hours or up to 12 hours if time permits.

2 Preheat the oven to 150°C (300°F/Gas 2). Put the bacon in a large heavy-based pan of water, bring to the boil, and blanch for 5 minutes. Drain and rinse with cold water. Remove the lamb from the marinade and dry on kitchen paper. Strain the marinade, reserving the liquid, bay leaf, and zest.

3 Put the bacon on the bottom of a large casserole and cover with the lamb. Layer the tomatoes and onions on top, then the carrots, mushrooms, and olives. Pour in the strained marinade and stock, season with pepper, and add the bay leaf and zest. Bring to the boil, cover with the lid, and put in the oven for 3½–4 hours. Check occasionally that it's not drying out, topping up with a little hot water if needed. Remove the bay leaf and zest, taste, and season if needed. Serve with mashed potatoes.

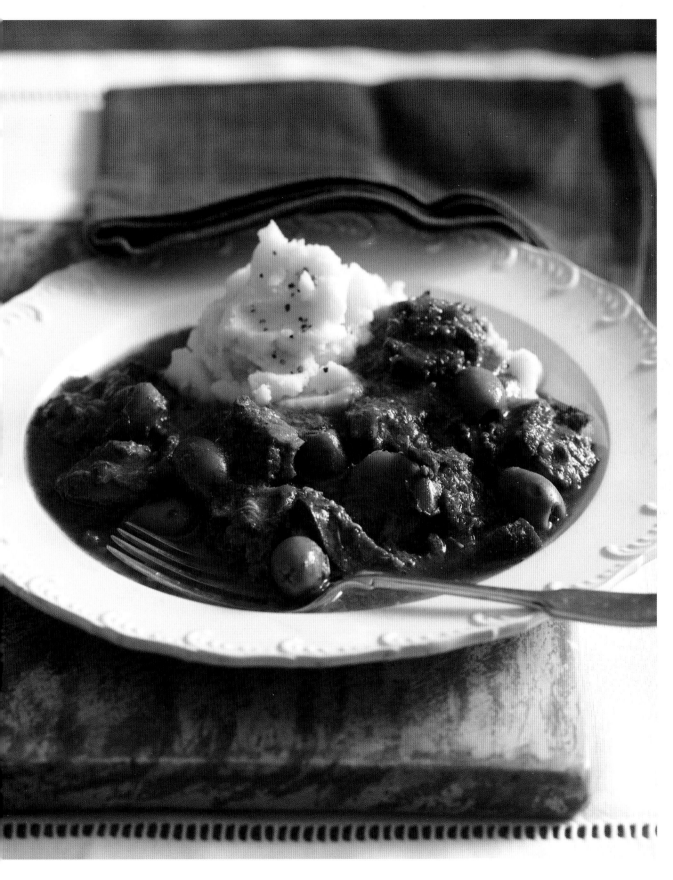

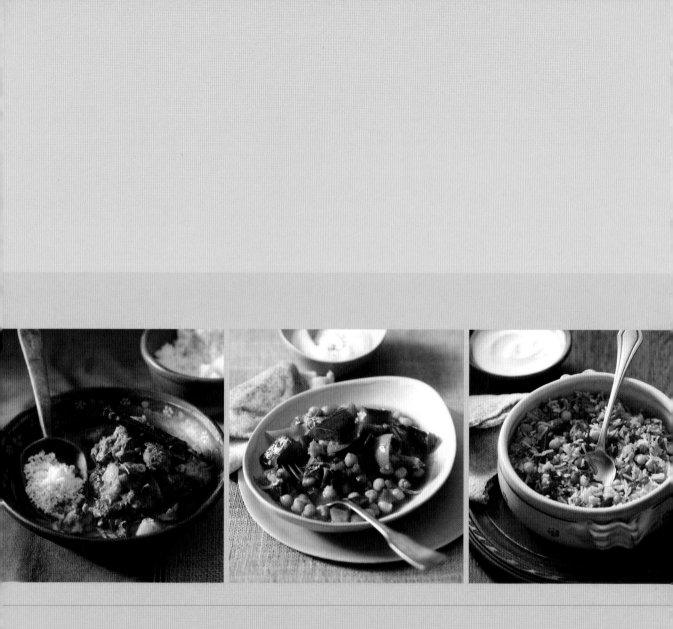

Tagines

This dish is slow cooked in a casserole, but you could always use a tagine if you have one. Preserved lemons have a subtle and distinctive flavour and are available at larger supermarkets.

Chicken and green olive tagine

SERVES 4–6   **FREEZE** UP TO 1 MONTH

4 tbsp olive oil
1 tbsp ground ginger
2 tbsp paprika
pinch of cayenne pepper
1 tsp ground turmeric
salt and freshly ground black pepper
8 chicken drumsticks
4 onions, roughly chopped
4 garlic cloves, finely chopped
pinch of saffron threads
2.5cm (1in) piece of fresh root ginger,
  peeled and grated

4 large tomatoes, roughly chopped
juice of ½ lemon for the slow cooker
  (1 lemon for the traditional method)
600ml (1 pint) hot vegetable stock for
  the slow cooker (900ml/1½ pints for
  the traditional method)
150g (5½oz) green olives in brine, stoned
  and rinsed
2 preserved lemons, halved, flesh discarded,
  and rind shredded (optional)
handful of coriander, chopped
handful of flat-leaf parsley, chopped

in the slow cooker   **PREP** 20 MINS, PLUS MARINATING   **COOK** 15 MINS PRECOOKING; **AUTO/LOW** 6–8 HRS OR **HIGH** 3–4 HRS

1 Preheat the slow cooker, if required. In a bowl, mix together half the oil with the spices and season with salt and pepper. Add the chicken drumsticks and toss until they are really well coated. Cover and leave overnight in the fridge, if time allows, or leave for 30 minutes. Heat a large flameproof casserole or tagine, add the chicken drumsticks (in batches and with extra oil, if necessary), and cook for 6–8 minutes until golden. Remove from the casserole and set aside.

2 Heat 1 tbsp of the oil in the casserole over a medium heat, add the onion, and cook for 3–4 minutes until soft. Then stir through the garlic, saffron, and grated ginger and cook for a minute more. Transfer everything to the slow cooker and add the tomatoes, chicken, lemon juice, stock, olives, and the preserved lemons, if using. Season, cover with the lid, and cook on auto/low for 6–8 hours or on high for 3–4 hours. Sprinkle over the herbs and serve with couscous.

traditional method   **PREP** 20 MINS, PLUS MARINATING   **COOK** 2 HRS

1 In a bowl, mix together half the oil with the spices and season with salt and pepper. Add the chicken drumsticks and toss until they are really well coated. Cover and leave overnight in the fridge, if time allows, or leave for 30 minutes. Preheat the oven to 190°C (375°F/Gas 5). Heat a large flameproof casserole or tagine, add the chicken drumsticks (in batches and with extra oil, if necessary), and cook for 6–8 minutes until golden. Remove from the casserole and set aside.

2 Heat 1 tbsp of the oil in the casserole, add the onion, and cook for 3–4 minutes until soft. Then stir through the garlic, grated ginger, and saffron and cook for a minute more. Stir in the tomatoes and return the chicken to the casserole with any juices and the lemon juice. Season and pour in the stock. Bring to the boil, then reduce to a simmer, cover, and put in the oven for 1 hour. Add the olives and preserved lemons, if using, and cook for 30 minutes more. Check occasionally that it's not drying out, topping up with a little hot water if needed. Sprinkle over the herbs and serve with couscous.

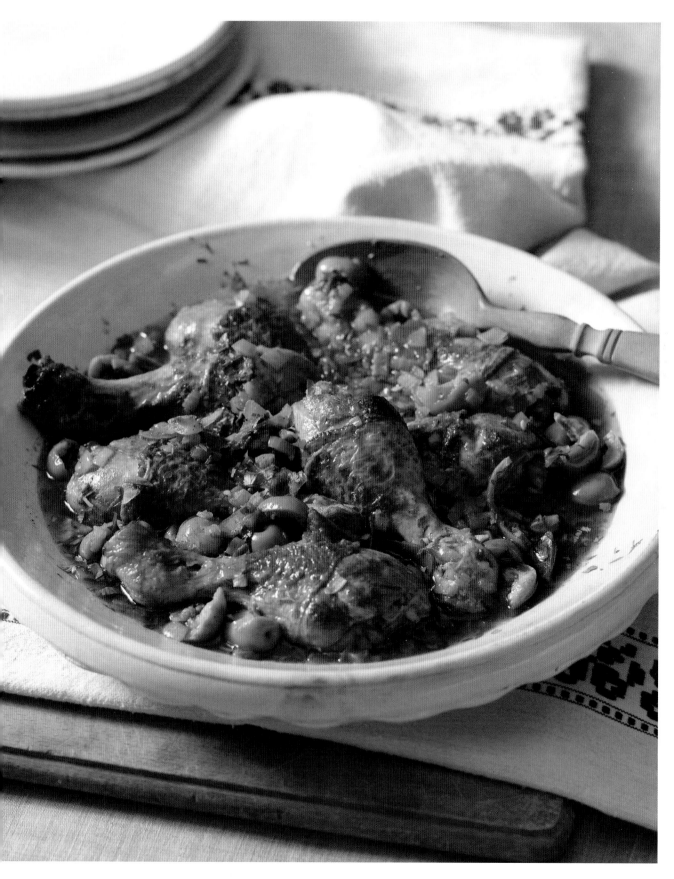

Chickpeas are a typical Middle Eastern ingredient. If you have the dried type, soak them in water for at least eight hours. Strain through a sieve, then rinse them under cold running water.

Middle Eastern lentils and peppers

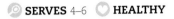 **SERVES** 4–6 **HEALTHY**

100g (3½oz) brown or green lentils, rinsed
salt and freshly ground black pepper
1 tbsp olive oil
1 onion, finely chopped
3 garlic cloves, finely chopped
pinch of dried oregano
grated zest and juice of 1 lemon
½ tsp ground allspice

pinch of grated nutmeg
½ tsp ground cumin
2 red peppers, deseeded and sliced into strips
200g (7oz) rice
600ml (1 pint) hot vegetable stock for the slow
 cooker (900ml/1½ pints for the traditional method)
400g can chickpeas, drained and rinsed
bunch of parsley, finely chopped

in the slow cooker **PREP** 15 MINS **COOK** 20 MINS PRECOOKING; **HIGH** 1½–2 HRS

1 Put the lentils in a large heavy-based pan or tagine, season with salt and pepper, and cover with water. Bring to the boil, then simmer for about 30 minutes until they are beginning to soften, but don't let them turn mushy. Drain and set aside.

2 Preheat the slow cooker, if required. Heat the oil in the same heavy-based pan over a medium heat, add the onion, and cook for 3–4 minutes until soft. Add seasoning, then stir through the garlic, oregano, lemon zest, allspice, nutmeg, and cumin and cook for a minute. Add the peppers and cook for about 5 minutes, stirring to coat with the spices. Cook for 2–3 minutes until soft, then stir in the rice and a little stock, and bring to the boil. Transfer everything to the slow cooker with the chickpeas and just enough stock to cover. Add the lid and cook on high for 1½–2 hours.

3 About 5 minutes before the end of the cooking time, stir through the lentils, put the lid back on, and let the lentils warm through. Taste and season, then add the parsley and lemon juice. Serve with yogurt and pitta bread.

traditional method **PREP** 15 MINS **COOK** 45 MINS

1 Put the lentils in a large heavy-based pan or tagine, season with salt and pepper, and cover with water. Bring to the boil, then simmer for about 30 minutes until they are beginning to soften, but don't let them turn mushy. Drain and set aside.

2 Meanwhile, heat the oil in another heavy-based pan over a medium heat, add the onion, and cook for 3–4 minutes until soft. Add seasoning, then stir through the garlic, oregano, lemon zest, allspice, nutmeg, and cumin and cook for a minute.

3 Add the peppers and cook for about 5 minutes, stirring to coat with spices. Cook for 2–3 minutes until soft, then stir in the rice and little stock. Bring to the boil, add most of the stock, and boil for a minute. Reduce to a simmer, add the chickpeas, and cook on a very low heat for 15–20 minutes. Check occasionally that it's not drying out, topping up with a little hot stock if needed. Stir through the lentils, taste and season, then add the parsley and lemon juice. Serve with yogurt and pitta bread.

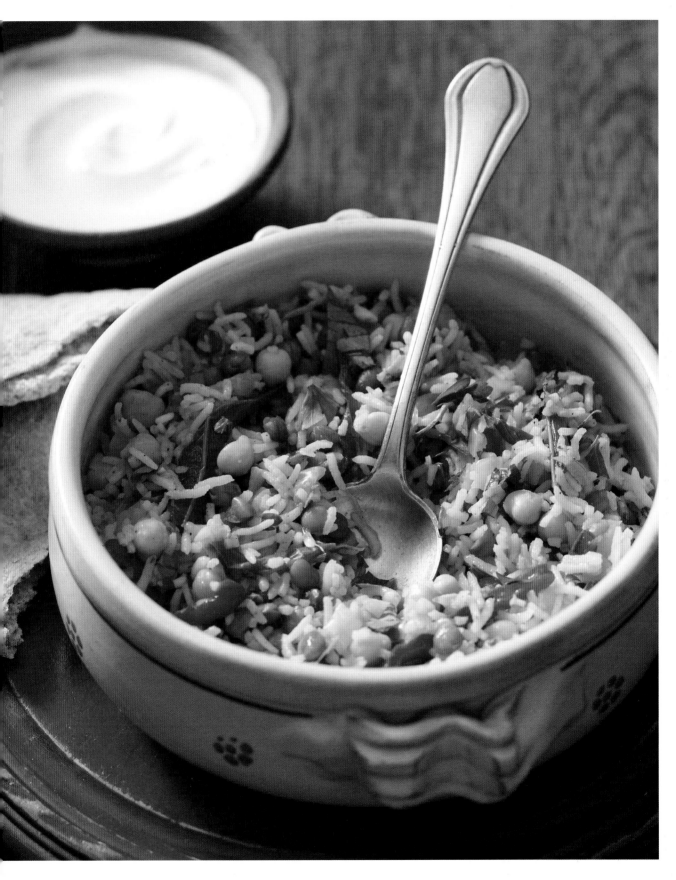

Hearty chestnuts give substance to this otherwise traditional combination of lamb and orange. The tagine tastes even better reheated the next day as the flavours will have melded together.

Slow-cooked lamb with orange and chestnuts

SERVES 4–6 **FREEZE** UP TO 1 MONTH

½ tsp ground cinnamon
½ tsp ground cumin
½ tsp ground coriander
salt and freshly ground black pepper
900g (2lb) lean leg of lamb, diced
2–3 tbsp olive oil
1 onion, chopped

1 cinnamon stick
175g (6oz) ready-cooked chestnuts
150ml (5fl oz) fresh orange juice
600ml (1 pint) hot lamb stock for the slow cooker
  (900ml/1½ pints for the traditional method)
2 oranges, peeled and cut into thick slices
bunch of coriander, roughly chopped

in the slow cooker **PREP** 15 MINS **COOK** 15–25 MINS PRECOOKING; AUTO/LOW 6–8 HRS

1 Preheat the slow cooker, if required. In a large bowl, mix together the spices and season with salt and pepper, then toss the meat in the mixture. Heat half the oil in a large flameproof casserole or tagine over a medium-high heat, add the lamb (in batches and with extra oil, if necessary), and cook for 6–8 minutes or until the lamb is browned on all sides. Remove and put in the slow cooker.

2 Heat the remaining oil in the casserole over a medium heat. Add the onion and cinnamon stick, and stir so the onion is coated in any residual lamb juices. Cook for 3–4 minutes until the onions are soft. Then stir in the chestnuts and pour in the orange juice. Increase the heat and let it bubble for a minute, stirring. Transfer everything to the slow cooker and pour in the stock. Cover and cook on auto/low for 6–8 hours. Add the orange slices for the last 30 minutes of cooking. Check for seasoning, stir through the coriander, and serve with couscous.

traditional method **PREP** 15 MINS **COOK** 2¼ HRS

1 Preheat the oven to 160°C (325°F/Gas 3). In a large bowl, mix together the spices and season with salt and pepper, then toss the meat in the mixture. Heat half the oil in a large flameproof casserole or tagine over a medium-high heat, add the lamb (in batches and with extra oil, if necessary), and cook for 6–8 minutes or until the lamb is browned on all sides. Remove and set aside.

2 Heat the remaining oil in the casserole over a medium heat. Add the onion and cinnamon stick, and stir so the onion is coated in any residual lamb juices. Cook for 3–4 minutes until the onions are soft. Then stir in the chestnuts and pour in the orange juice. Increase the heat and let it bubble for a minute, stirring. Reduce the heat and return the lamb to the casserole along with any juices from the lamb.

3 Pour in the stock, bring to the boil, then reduce to a simmer, cover, and put in the oven for 2 hours. Check occasionally that it's not drying out, topping up with a little hot water, if needed. Add the orange slices for the last 30 minutes of cooking. Check for seasoning, stir through the coriander, and serve with couscous.

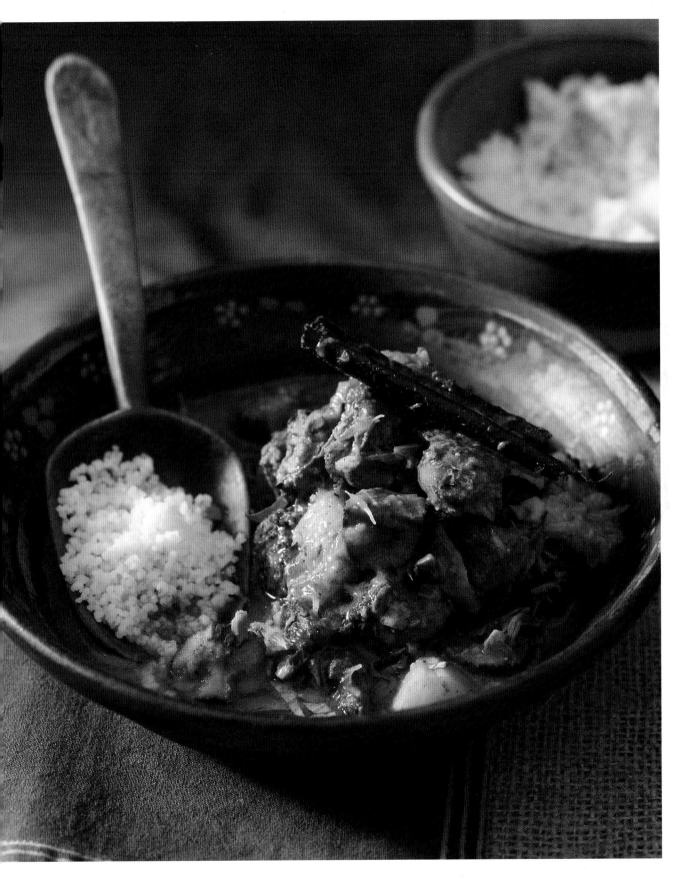

One of the spices in this recipe is sumac, a Middle Eastern spice that is slightly tart in taste. It is found in most major supermarkets. Black olives are suggested, but use green if you prefer.

Red mullet with Middle Eastern spices

SERVES 4–6 **FREEZE** UP TO 1 MONTH **HEALTHY**

1 tbsp olive oil
6 shallots, finely chopped
1 fennel bulb, trimmed and finely chopped
1 carrot, peeled and finely chopped
½ tsp ground cumin
1 tsp of sumac or use a preserved lemon, flesh discarded and rind finely chopped (optional)
4 plum tomatoes, roughly chopped
600ml (1 pint) hot vegetable stock for the slow cooker (900ml/1½ pints for the traditional method)

salt and freshly ground black pepper
8 black olives, stoned
about 1.6kg (3½lb) red mullet, filleted (about 675g/1½lb filleted weight) and cut into chunky pieces
small handful of coriander, finely chopped
small handful of mint, finely chopped
1 preserved lemon, flesh discarded and rind sliced finely, to serve (optional)

in the slow cooker **PREP** 15 MINS **COOK** 10 MINS PRECOOKING; **HIGH** 3–4 HRS

1 Preheat the slow cooker, if required. Heat the oil in a large heavy-based pan or tagine over a medium heat, add the shallots, fennel, and carrot, and cook for 5 minutes until soft. Stir through the cumin and sumac or preserved lemon, and cook for a further minute.

2 Transfer everything to the slow cooker, then stir through the tomatoes and just enough stock to cover the vegetables, and season with salt and pepper. Add the olives, cover with the lid, and cook on high for 3–4 hours, adding the fish for the last 30 minutes of cooking.

3 Stir through most of the coriander and mint, taste and season, if needed. Serve with couscous and scatter over the remaining fresh herbs and preserved lemon rind, if using.

traditional method **PREP** 15 MINS **COOK** 1½ HRS

1 Heat the oil in a large heavy-based pan or tagine, add the shallots, fennel, and carrot, and cook for 5 minutes until soft. Stir through the cumin and sumac or preserved lemon, and cook for a further minute. Add the tomatoes and stock, season with salt and pepper, and bring to the boil, then reduce to a simmer.

2 Add the olives, partially cover with a lid, and simmer gently for about 1 hour, stirring occasionally and topping up with hot water, if needed. Sit the fish on top of the tomato mixture, cover with the lid, and cook for a further 10 minutes or until the fish is cooked through.

3 Stir through most of the coriander and mint, taste and season, if needed. Serve with couscous and scatter over the remaining fresh herbs and preserved lemon rind, if using.

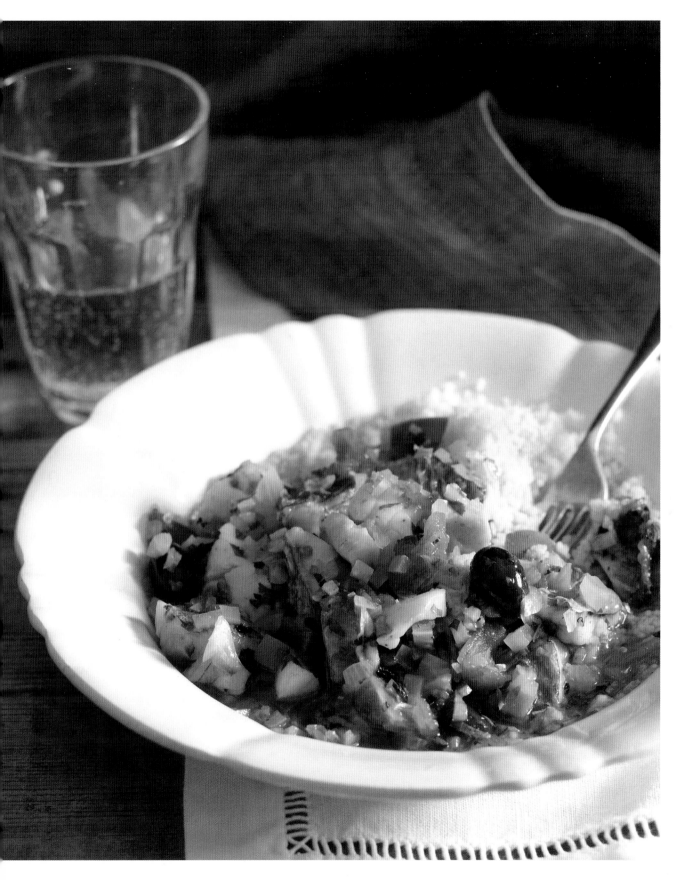

This is a vegetarian dish full of taste and texture with its fleshy aubergine and nutty chickpeas. It is an ideal dish to prepare a day ahead as the flavours become even better with time.

Middle Eastern chickpea stew

SERVES 4–6 **FREEZE** UP TO 3 MONTHS **HEALTHY**

2 tbsp olive oil
1 red onion, finely chopped
salt and freshly ground black pepper
½ tsp ground cinnamon
½ tsp ground cumin
½ tsp sumac (optional)
4 garlic cloves, finely chopped
1 large aubergine, roughly chopped into bite-sized pieces
150ml (5fl oz) white wine
2 x 400g cans chickpeas, drained and rinsed

400g can chopped tomatoes
1–2 tsp harissa paste, depending on how spicy you like it
60g (2oz) dried cherries or cranberries or use fresh pomegranate seeds
2 preserved lemons, quartered, flesh removed and discarded (optional)
600ml (1 pint) hot vegetable stock for the slow cooker (900ml/1½ pints for the traditional method)
bunch of coriander leaves, chopped

in the slow cooker PREP 10 MINS COOK 15 MINS PRECOOKING; AUTO/LOW 6–8 HRS OR HIGH 3–4 HRS

1 Preheat the slow cooker, if required. Heat the oil in a large heavy-based pan or tagine over a medium heat, add the onion, and cook for 3–4 minutes until soft. Season with salt and pepper, stir through the spices, garlic, and aubergine, and cook for 5–8 minutes, stirring, so it is all coated and the aubergine starts to turn golden brown.

2 Transfer everything to the slow cooker, then add the wine to the pan and stir to deglaze the residual pan juices before also transferring to the slow cooker. Add the chickpeas, tomatoes, harissa paste, cherries, preserved lemons (if using), and the stock. Season and stir, then cover with the lid, and cook on auto/low for 6–8 hours or on high for 3–4 hours.

3 Taste and season if needed, or stir through more harissa paste if you like it hot. Stir through most of the coriander and ladle into warmed shallow bowls, then sprinkle with the remaining coriander. Serve with warm flatbread and a spoonful of plain yogurt on the side.

traditional method PREP 10 MINS COOK 1¼ HRS

1 Heat the oil in a large heavy-based pan or tagine over a medium heat, add the onion, and cook for 3–4 minutes until soft. Season with salt and pepper, stir through the spices, garlic, and aubergine, and cook for 5–8 minutes, stirring, so it is all coated and the aubergine starts to turn golden brown.

2 Add the wine and let it bubble for a minute, then add the chickpeas, tomatoes, harissa paste, cherries, and preserved lemons, if using. Stir well and pour in the stock. Bring to the boil, then reduce to a simmer, partially cover with the lid, and cook gently for 1 hour, stirring occasionally.

3 Taste and season if needed, or stir through more harissa paste if you like it hot. Stir through most of the coriander and ladle into warmed shallow bowls, then sprinkle with the remaining coriander. Serve with warm flatbread and a spoonful of plain yogurt on the side.

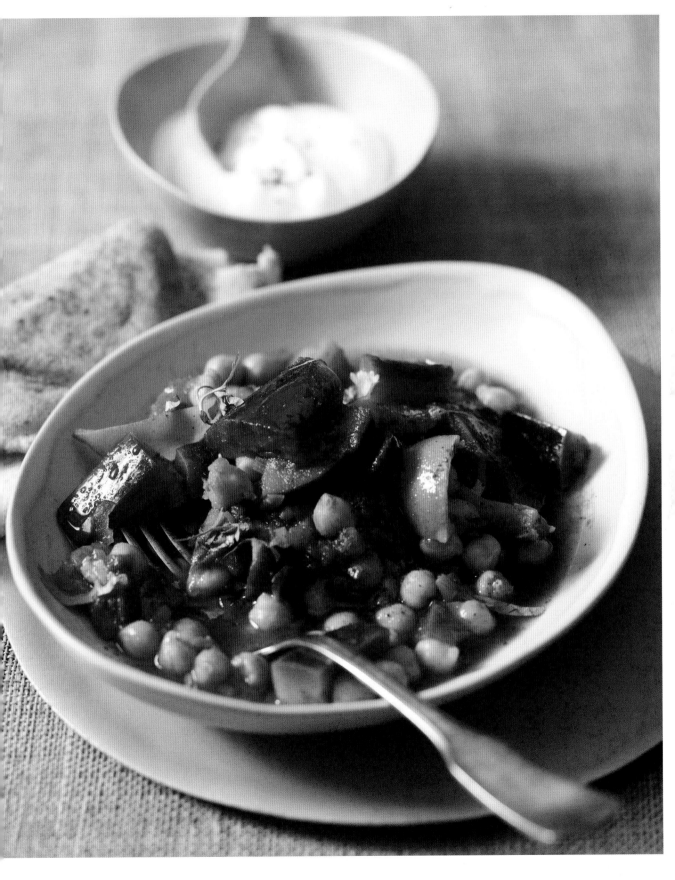

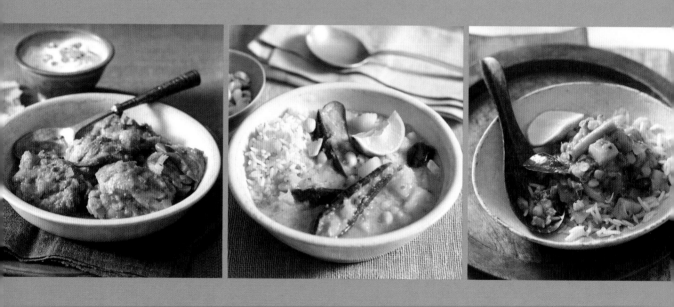

Curries

This is a relatively dry curry, although if you like a curry with more sauce, you can top up the stock during cooking. Fresh ginger and bird's eye chillies make the dish more fragrant.

Karahi chicken

⊚ **SERVES** 4 ⊛ **FREEZE** UP TO 1 MONTH ⬭ **HEALTHY**

1 tsp coriander seeds
2 green chillies, deseeded
3 garlic cloves, peeled
1 tsp ground turmeric
2 tbsp sunflower oil
8 chicken thighs, skin on, slashed a few
  times across each thigh
salt and freshly ground black pepper

1 onion, roughly chopped
6 tomatoes, roughly chopped
450ml (15fl oz) hot vegetable stock for the slow
  cooker (900ml/1½ pints for the traditional method)
5cm (2in) piece of fresh root ginger, peeled and
  finely chopped
3–4 green bird's eye chillies, left whole
bunch of coriander, finely chopped

in the slow cooker ⏱ **PREP** 15 MINS   **COOK** 25 MINS PRECOOKING;
AUTO/LOW 6 HRS OR HIGH 3 HRS

1 Preheat the slow cooker, if required. Put the coriander seeds, chillies, garlic, turmeric, and half the oil into a food processor and blend until it becomes a paste. Season the chicken with salt and pepper and smother them with the paste, using your hands and pushing it into all the cuts. Heat half the remaining oil in a large flameproof casserole over a medium-high heat and add the chicken pieces. Cook for 5–6 minutes on each side or until beginning to colour, then remove and set aside.

2 Heat the remaining oil in the casserole over a medium heat, add the onion, and cook for 3–4 minutes until soft. Then add the tomatoes and cook for 5–10 minutes until they, too, are soft. Transfer everything to the slow cooker. Pour over the stock and add the ginger, bird's eye chillies, and chicken, pushing the chicken under the liquid as much as you can. Cover with the lid and cook on auto/low for 6 hours or on high for 3 hours. Remove the chillies, then taste and season as necessary, stirring through the coriander. Serve with rice, chapatis, and some minted yogurt on the side.

traditional method ⏱ **PREP** 15 MINS   **COOK** 1 HR

1 Put the coriander seeds, chillies, garlic, turmeric, and half the oil into a food processor and blend until it becomes a paste. Season the chicken with salt and pepper and smother them with the paste, using your hands and pushing it into all the cuts. Heat half the remaining oil in a large flameproof casserole over a medium-high heat and add the chicken pieces. Cook for 5–6 minutes on each side or until beginning to colour, then remove and set aside.

2 Heat the remaining oil in the casserole over a medium heat, add the onion, and cook for 3–4 minutes until soft. Then add the tomatoes and cook for a further 5–10 minutes until they, too, are soft. Pour in the stock and bring to the boil. Reduce to a simmer, stir in the ginger and bird's eye chillies, and return the chicken to the casserole. Cover with the lid and cook gently for 30–40 minutes, keeping an eye on the sauce. You want it to be fairly dry, but if it is sticking, add a little hot water.

3 Remove the chillies, then taste and season, as necessary, stirring through the coriander. Serve with rice, chapatis, and some minted yogurt on the side.

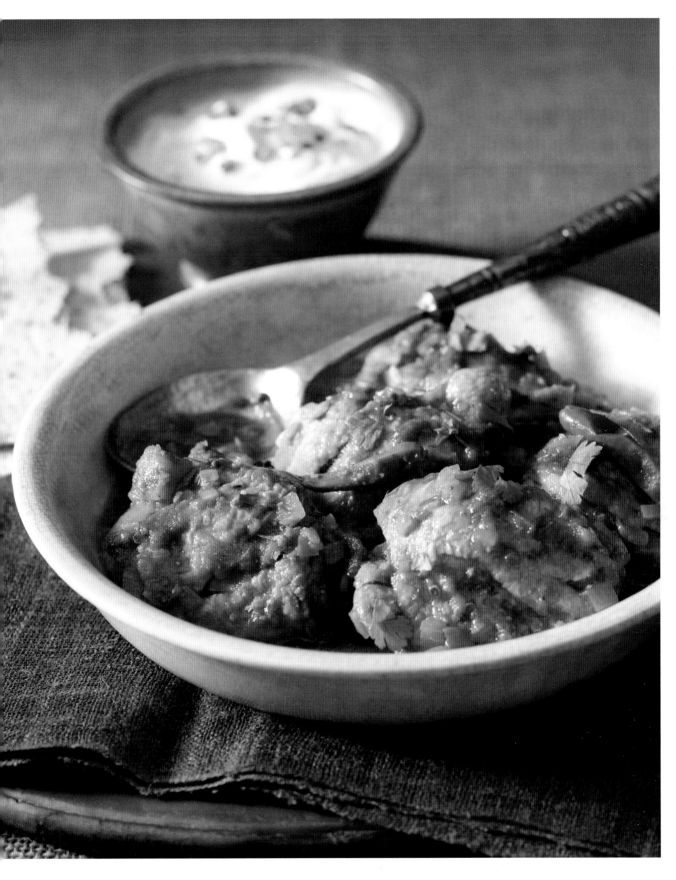

A classic Cambodian braised curry, this recipe has dominant cardamom and ginger flavours; the addition of peanuts helps to thicken the sauce. Serve with rice and pickled vegetables.

Cardamom and ginger beef curry

SERVES 4

675g (1½lb) boneless beef shin steak or thin flank, cut into 4cm (1½in) cubes

85g (3oz) fresh root ginger, finely grated and squeezed to extract the juice (discard the fibres)

3 tbsp vegetable oil

1 tbsp shrimp paste

400ml can coconut milk

4 tbsp palm sugar or granulated sugar

1 tbsp tamarind paste mixed with 4 tbsp water

2 tbsp fish sauce (nam pla)

75g (2½oz) unsalted roasted peanut halves

2–4 red Thai chillies, deseeded and thinly sliced (optional)

FOR THE CURRY PASTE

2 tbsp sunflower oil

3 dried red chillies, soaked, deseeded and halved

4 large garlic cloves, crushed

1 large shallot, coarsely chopped

1 stalk lemongrass, trimmed and sliced

7.5cm (3in) piece cinnamon stick

2 star anise

7 cardamom pods, crushed

1 tsp grated nutmeg

½ tsp ground mace

1½ tbsp finely chopped coriander

¼ tsp ground turmeric

in the slow cooker

PREP 20 MINS, PLUS MARINATING
COOK 15 MINS PRECOOKING; AUTO/LOW 5–6 HRS OR HIGH 3–4 HRS

1 In a bowl, combine the beef with the ginger juice, tossing to coat. Leave to marinate for 30 minutes. To make the curry paste, heat the oil in a flameproof casserole over a moderate heat and stir-fry the chillies, garlic, shallot, and lemongrass until fragrant. Add the spices (except coriander and turmeric) and stir-fry for 5–7 minutes until toasted. Transfer to a food processor, add the coriander and turmeric, and blend until smooth, adding water (1 tbsp at a time, as necessary) to ease the process. Set the paste aside.

2 Preheat the slow cooker, if required. Heat the oil in the casserole over a moderate heat and briefly stir-fry the shrimp paste. Add the curry paste and half the coconut milk. Stir, transfer to the slow cooker, and add the beef. Stir in the remaining coconut milk, sugar, tamarind water, fish sauce, and nuts. Cover and cook on auto/low for 5–6 hours or on high for 3–4 hours. Serve with Thai chillies, if using.

traditional method

PREP 20 MINS, PLUS MARINATING **COOK** 2–2¼ HRS

1 In a bowl, combine the beef with the ginger juice, tossing to coat. Leave to marinate for 30 minutes. To make the curry paste, heat the oil in a flameproof casserole over a moderate heat and stir-fry the chillies, garlic, shallot, and lemongrass until fragrant. Add the spices (except coriander and turmeric) and stir-fry for 5–7 minutes until toasted. Transfer to a food processor, add the coriander and turmeric, and blend until smooth, adding water (1 tbsp at a time, as necessary) to ease the process. Set the paste aside.

2 Heat the oil in the casserole over a moderate heat and briefly stir-fry the shrimp paste. Add the curry paste and half the coconut milk. Stir, then add the beef. Cook for 20 minutes, stirring occasionally. Reduce the heat to low and stir in the remaining coconut milk, sugar, tamarind water, fish sauce, and nuts. Season with salt, if needed. Simmer, covered, for 1½–2 hours or until the meat is fork tender, adding more coconut milk if the stew thickens too much. Serve with Thai chillies, if using.

An intensely flavoured Indonesian speciality, originally made with water buffalo. It can be made up to 2 days ahead and kept in the refrigerator. Bring to room temperature, then reheat on the stove.

Beef rendang

SERVES 6

2 x 400ml cans coconut milk (3 x 400ml cans for the traditional method)
4 bay leaves
1.35kg (3lb) beef chuck steak, cut in 5cm (2in) cubes
salt

FOR THE CURRY PASTE
2.5cm (1in) piece cinnamon stick, ground or pounded
12 cloves, ground or pounded
2 stalks lemongrass, trimmed and roughly chopped
6 shallots, quartered
7.5cm (3in) piece fresh root ginger, roughly chopped
6 garlic cloves, peeled and left whole
6 red chillies, deseeded and roughly chopped
1 tsp ground turmeric

in the slow cooker
PREP 15 MINS **COOK** 10 MINS PRECOOKING; AUTO/LOW 6–8 HRS

1 Preheat the slow cooker, if required. Put all the ingredients for the curry paste in a food processor and whiz to make a thick paste. If the mixture is very thick, add about 4 tbsp of the coconut milk. Transfer the curry paste to a wok or large heavy-based pan, add the coconut milk, and stir until well mixed. Add the bay leaves and bring to the boil over a high heat, stirring occasionally.

2 Transfer the coconut sauce to the slow cooker together with the beef and season with salt. Cover with the lid and cook on auto/low for 6–8 hours.

3 Taste the curry and add more salt if needed. Spoon the curried beef onto a bed of cooked rice on warmed plates or in shallow bowls.

traditional method
PREP 15 MINS **COOK** 3¾ –4¼ HRS

1 Put all the ingredients for the curry paste in a food processor and whiz to make a thick paste. If the mixture is very thick, add about 4 tbsp of the coconut milk. Transfer the curry paste to a wok or large heavy-based pan, add the coconut milk, and stir until well mixed. Add the bay leaves and bring to the boil over a high heat, stirring occasionally.

2 Reduce the heat to medium and cook the sauce, stirring occasionally, for about 15 minutes. Add the beef and salt, stir, and bring to the boil. Reduce the heat to medium and simmer, uncovered, stirring occasionally, for 2 hours.

3 Reduce the heat to very low and continue cooking for 1½–2 hours, partially covered, until the beef is tender and the sauce quite thick. Stir frequently to prevent sticking. Skim off all the fat, taste the curry, and add more salt if needed. It will be very thick and rich. Towards the end of cooking, oil will separate from the sauce and the beef will fry in it. Spoon the curried beef onto a bed of cooked rice on warmed plates or in shallow bowls.

This is a great vegetarian dish, with distinctively sweet flavours of cinnamon and cardamom. The peanuts add a contrasting texture to the potatoes and aubergine. Make it as hot and fiery as you wish.

Aubergine massaman curry

SERVES 4–6

2 red chillies, deseeded
1 lemongrass stalk, tough outer leaves removed
5cm (2in) piece of fresh root ginger, peeled and roughly chopped
5 cardamom pods, crushed
1 tbsp sunflower oil
1 onion, finely chopped
salt and freshly ground black pepper
450ml (15fl oz) hot vegetable stock for the slow cooker (600ml/1 pint for the traditional method)
400ml can coconut milk

1 cinnamon stick, broken
splash of dark soy sauce
splash of fish sauce (nam pla) – omit if cooking for vegetarians
4 potatoes, peeled and chopped into bite-sized pieces
6 baby aubergines, halved lengthways, or use 2 large ones, roughly chopped
1 tbsp palm sugar or demerara sugar (optional)
85g (3oz) roasted unsalted peanuts, roughly chopped

in the slow cooker **PREP** 15 MINS **COOK** 15 MINS PRECOOKING; AUTO/LOW 8 HRS OR HIGH 3–4 HRS

1 Preheat the slow cooker, if required. Put the chillies, lemongrass, ginger, and cardamom in a food processor and whiz with a drop of the sunflower oil to make a paste.

2 Heat the remaining oil in a large heavy-based pan over a medium heat, add the onion, and cook for 3–4 minutes until soft. Then add the paste and some seasoning and cook for a few minutes more. Stir in the stock and coconut milk and bring to the boil, then add the cinnamon stick, soy sauce, and fish sauce, if using, and stir. Reduce to a simmer and leave uncovered for about 20 minutes, for the sauce to thicken slightly. Transfer everything to the slow cooker and add the potatoes and aubergines. Cover with the lid and cook on auto/low for 8 hours or on high for 3–4 hours.

3 Taste and season with the sugar, if using, and stir in half the peanuts. Ladle into warmed bowls and sprinkle with the remaining peanuts. Serve with rice and lime wedges.

traditional method **PREP** 15 MINS **COOK** 1 HR

1 Put the chillies, lemongrass, ginger, and cardamom in a food processor and whiz with a drop of the sunflower oil to make a paste.

2 Heat the remaining oil in a large heavy-based pan over a medium heat, add the onion, and cook for 3–4 minutes until soft. Then add the paste and some seasoning and cook for a few minutes more. Stir in the stock and coconut milk, and bring to the boil, then add the cinnamon stick, soy sauce, and fish sauce, if using, and cook on a low heat for about 20 minutes. Stir in the potatoes and aubergines and cook for a further 20 minutes.

3 Stir in half the peanuts, taste, and adjust the flavour by adding the sugar, if using, and more salt or fish sauce, also if using, as needed. Ladle into warmed bowls and sprinkle with the remaining peanuts. Serve with rice and lime wedges.

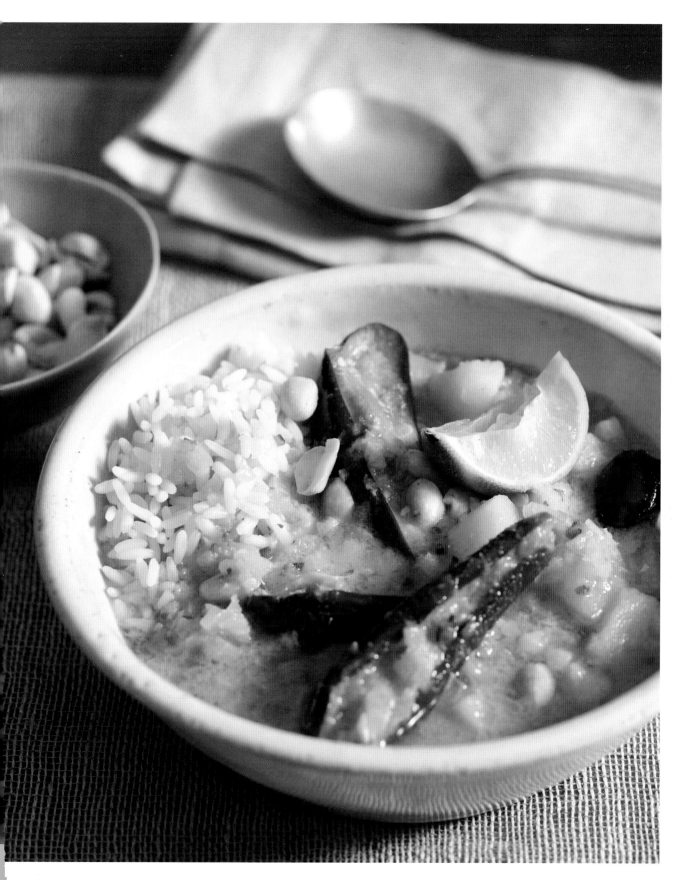

Prawns need minimal cooking, so they can simply be stirred through at the end. You could use ready-cooked ones instead, if you prefer, or you could stir though some cooked chicken.

Prawn makhani

SERVES 4–6   **FREEZE** UP TO 3 MONTHS, WITHOUT THE CREAM

3 tbsp vegetable oil
3 garlic cloves, finely chopped
5cm (2in) piece of fresh root ginger, peeled
  and finely chopped
1 cinnamon stick, broken into pieces
2 red chillies, deseeded and finely chopped
4 cardamom pods, crushed
500g (1lb 2oz) tomatoes, chopped

700g (1lb 9oz) (shelled weight) uncooked prawns
salt and freshly ground black pepper
200ml (7fl oz) thick plain yogurt
1–2 tsp medium-hot chilli powder
75g (2½oz) cashew nuts, ground, plus a handful,
  roughly chopped, to serve
1–2 tsp ground fenugreek
100ml (3½fl oz) double cream

in the slow cooker   **PREP** 20 MINS, PLUS MARINATING   **COOK** 10 MINS PRECOOKING; **AUTO/LOW** 4–5 HRS OR **HIGH** 3–4 HRS

1 Preheat the slow cooker, if required. Heat 2 tbsp of the oil in a large heavy-based pan over a low heat, add half the garlic, half the ginger, the cinnamon, chillies, and cardamom pods and cook, stirring occasionally, for 2 minutes. Stir in the tomatoes and 100ml (3½fl oz) of water. Transfer everything to the slow cooker, cover with the lid, and cook on auto/low for 4–5 hours or on high for 3–4 hours.

2 At the last hour of cooking, season the prawns with salt and pepper and toss with the rest of the garlic and ginger, the remaining oil, the yogurt, and chilli powder. Leave to marinate for 20 minutes. Meanwhile, use a stick blender to whiz the mixture in the slow cooker until smooth, stir in the ground cashews and fenugreek, and continue cooking.

3 Heat the pan over a high heat, then add the prawns and yogurt marinade and cook, tossing them all the time, for 5–8 minutes until no longer pink. For the last 5 minutes of cooking, add the prawns and cream to the slow cooker. Season if needed. Garnish with the chopped cashews and serve with rice.

traditional method   **PREP** 20 MINS, PLUS MARINATING   **COOK** 40 MINS

1 Heat 2 tbsp of the oil in a large heavy-based pan over a low heat, add half the garlic, half the ginger, the cinnamon, chillies, and cardamom pods and cook, stirring occasionally, for 2 minutes. Stir in the tomatoes and cook for 10 minutes or until they start to reduce. Cover with a little hot water and simmer for a further 10 minutes or until puréed. Push the tomato mixture through a sieve into a food processor and whiz until smooth.

2 Season the prawns with salt and pepper and toss with the rest of the garlic and ginger, the remaining oil, the yogurt, and chilli powder. Leave to marinate for 20 minutes. Heat the pan over a high heat, then add the prawns and yogurt marinade and cook, tossing them all the time, for 5–8 minutes until no longer pink. Remove and set aside.

3 Return the tomatoes to the pan, stir in the ground cashews and fenugreek, and simmer for 10 minutes, adding a little hot water if the sauce looks too thick. For the last 5 minutes of cooking, add the prawns and cream. Season if needed. Garnish with the chopped cashews and serve with rice.

Traditionally, dhansak would be made with three different types of lentils and plenty of vegetables. This version is simpler, but no less tasty for that. It can be made two days ahead and reheated.

Lamb dhansak

⊙ **SERVES** 6   ❄ **FREEZE** UP TO 3 MONTHS

4 tbsp vegetable oil
750g (1lb 10oz) boned shoulder of lamb, cut into
   bite-sized pieces
salt and freshly ground black pepper
1 large aubergine, chopped into bite-sized pieces
1 large onion, finely chopped
2cm (¾in) piece of fresh root ginger, peeled
   and finely chopped

5 garlic cloves, finely chopped
2 tsp ground cumin
2 tsp ground coriander
2 tsp ground turmeric
pinch of cayenne pepper
1 tbsp plain flour
175g (6oz) green lentils
1 small cauliflower, chopped into florets

in the slow cooker   ⏱ **PREP** 20 MINS   **COOK** 20 MINS PRECOOKING;
                                                          AUTO/LOW 6–8 HRS OR **HIGH** 3–4 HRS

1 Preheat the slow cooker, if required. Heat two-thirds of the oil in a large flameproof casserole over a high heat. Season the lamb with salt and pepper and cook (in batches, if necessary), stirring, for 3–5 minutes until brown on all sides. Remove and set aside. Add the remaining oil to the casserole, then add the aubergine and cook over a medium heat, stirring occasionally, for 5–7 minutes until brown. Also remove and set aside, but in a separate bowl.

2 Add the onion to the casserole and cook for 7–10 minutes until golden brown. Stir in the ginger and garlic and cook for 2–3 minutes until softened and fragrant. Add the ground cumin, coriander, turmeric, and cayenne, and cook for 1–2 minutes until thoroughly combined. Return the lamb with any juices, sprinkle with the flour, and cook, stirring, for about 1 minute. Stir in 450ml (15fl oz) of water and bring to the boil. Transfer everything to the slow cooker, then stir in the lentils. Cover with the lid and cook on auto/low for 6–8 hours or on high for 3–4 hours. Stir in the aubergine and cauliflower for the last 30 minutes of cooking, topping up with water if necessary. Serve with fluffy rice and a mango chutney.

traditional method   ⏱ **PREP** 20 MINS   **COOK** 2 HRS

1 Heat two-thirds of the oil in a large flameproof casserole over a high heat. Season the lamb with salt and pepper and cook (in batches, if necessary), stirring, for 3–5 minutes until brown on all sides. Remove and set aside. Add the remaining oil to the casserole, then add the aubergine and cook over a medium heat, stirring occasionally, for 5–7 minutes until brown. Also remove and set aside, but in a separate bowl.

2 Add the onion to the casserole and cook for 7–10 minutes until golden brown. Stir in the ginger and garlic and cook for 2–3 minutes until softened and fragrant. Add the ground cumin, coriander, turmeric, and cayenne, and cook for 1–2 minutes until thoroughly combined. Return the lamb with any juices, sprinkle with the flour, and cook, stirring, for about 1 minute. Stir in 1 litre (1¾ pints) of water and bring to the boil. Lower the heat, cover, and simmer gently, stirring occasionally, for 30 minutes. Stir in the lentils and cook for 15 minutes longer. Stir in the aubergine, cauliflower, and 500ml (16fl oz) more water; continue simmering, stirring often, for 50–60 minutes until completely tender. Add more water during cooking if the curry seems dry. Serve with fluffy rice and a mango chutney.

Duck curry is extremely rich and has a great depth of flavour. If you like your curry hot, use two red chillies rather than the one specified – and leave the seeds in for an even greater kick.

Duck curry

SERVES 4   **FREEZE** UP TO 1 MONTH

2 duck breasts
1 tbsp sunflower oil
1 onion, finely chopped
2 celery sticks, finely chopped
salt and freshly ground black pepper
3 garlic cloves, finely chopped
1 red chilli, deseeded and finely chopped
5cm (2in) piece of fresh root ginger, peeled
  and finely chopped

2 carrots, peeled and finely chopped
1 tbsp garam masala
1 tsp ground turmeric
1 tsp paprika
1 tbsp tomato purée
2 x 400g cans chopped tomatoes
600ml (1 pint) hot vegetable stock
  for the slow cooker (900ml/1½ pints
  for the traditional method)

in the slow cooker   PREP 15 MINS   COOK 25 MINS PRECOOKING; AUTO/LOW 8 HRS

1 Preheat the slow cooker, if required. Heat a heavy-based pan over a medium-high heat and add the duck breasts, skin-side down. Cook each side for 3–6 minutes until golden. Remove and set aside. Heat the oil in the pan over a medium heat, add the onion and celery, and cook for about 5 minutes until soft. Season with salt and pepper, stir in the garlic, chilli, and ginger, and cook for a couple more minutes. Add the carrots, turn to coat, and continue cooking for 5 more minutes, stirring occasionally. Stir through the spices and tomato purée and cook for 1–2 minutes.

2 Transfer everything to the slow cooker and then add the tomatoes and stock. Add the duck breasts and tuck them into the sauce. Cover with the lid and cook on auto/low for 8 hours. Remove the duck breasts, peel off the skin, and then shred the meat. Put the duck meat back into the slow cooker and stir, then taste and season, as required. Serve with rice and chapatis.

traditional method   PREP 15 MINS   COOK 2 HRS

1 Preheat the oven to 180°C (350°F/Gas 4). Heat a large flameproof casserole over a medium-high heat and add the duck breasts, skin-side down. Cook each side for 3–6 minutes or until golden. Remove and set aside. Heat the oil in the casserole over a medium heat, add the onion and celery, and cook for about 5 minutes until soft. Season with salt and pepper, stir in the garlic, chilli, and ginger, and cook for a couple more minutes.

2 Add the carrots, turn to coat, and continue cooking for 5 more minutes, stirring occasionally. Stir through the spices and tomato purée and cook for 1–2 minutes, then tip in the tomatoes and stock. Bring to the boil, reduce to a simmer, and return the duck breasts to the casserole, tucking them into the sauce. Cover with the lid and put in the oven for 1½ hours. Check occasionally that it's not drying out, topping up with a little hot water if needed.

3 Remove from the oven and spoon out the duck breasts. Peel off the skin and then shred the meat. Put the duck meat back into the casserole and return it to the oven for another 30 minutes (if the sauce is too thin, remove the lid). Taste and season, if necessary. Serve with rice and chapatis.

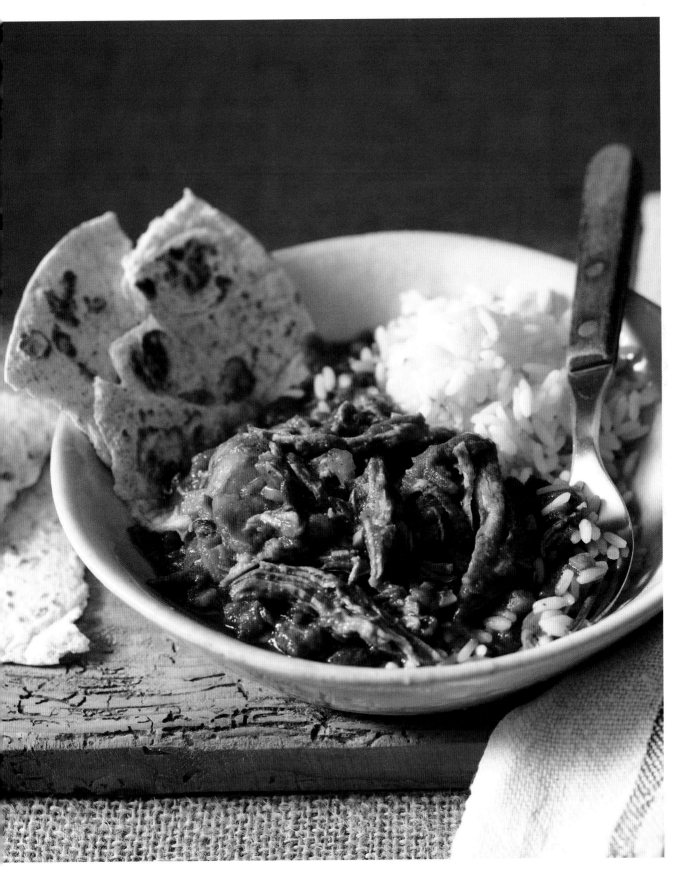

This is a hot and sour curry that features chillies and pineapple in a thick sauce of lentils, which successfully temper the heat and add texture to the finished dish.

Prawn dhansak

SERVES 6 **FREEZE** UP TO 3 MONTHS

250g (9oz) red lentils
salt and freshly ground black pepper
3 tbsp vegetable oil or 2 tbsp ghee
4 cardamom pods, crushed
2 tsp mustard seeds
2 tsp chilli powder
2 tsp ground turmeric
2 tsp ground cinnamon
2 onions, finely chopped

10cm (4in) piece fresh root ginger, peeled and finely chopped
4 garlic cloves, finely chopped
3–4 green chillies, deseeded and finely sliced
½ pineapple, peeled and cut into bite-sized pieces
6 tomatoes, skinned and roughly chopped
450g (1lb) (shelled weight) uncooked king prawns
handful of coriander, finely chopped

in the slow cooker
PREP 15 MINS **COOK** 10 MINS PRECOOKING;
AUTO/LOW 6–8 HRS OR **HIGH** 3–4 HRS

1 Preheat the slow cooker, if required. Put the lentils in the slow cooker, season well with salt and pepper, then pour in enough cold water to cover. Cover with the lid and cook on auto/low for 6–8 hours or on high for 3–4 hours.

2 While the lentils are starting to cook, heat 1 tbsp of the oil or ½ tbsp of the ghee in a large heavy-based pan, add the dried spices, and cook, stirring, for 2 minutes or until the seeds pop. Stir in the onions, ginger, garlic, and chillies, and cook for 5 minutes or until soft and fragrant. Transfer to the slow cooker with the lentils, re-cover with the lid, and continue cooking.

3 Heat 1 tbsp of the oil or ½ tbsp of ghee in the pan, stir through the pineapple and tomatoes, then stir these into the lentils for the last 30 minutes of cooking. When ready to serve, heat the remaining oil or ghee, add the prawns, and cook briefly until pink, then stir them into the lentils. Taste and season if needed, stir through the coriander, and serve with rice or naan bread.

traditional method
PREP 15 MINS **COOK** 50 MINS

1 Put the lentils in a large heavy-based pan, season well with salt and pepper, then pour in enough cold water to cover. Cover with the lid, bring to the boil, then reduce to a simmer, and cook for 20 minutes or until soft. Top up with hot water if they begin to dry out. Drain and set aside.

2 Meanwhile, heat 1 tbsp of the oil or ½ tbsp of the ghee in a large heavy-based pan, add the dried spices, and cook, stirring, for 2 minutes or until the seeds pop. Stir in the onions, ginger, garlic, and chillies, and cook for 5 minutes or until soft and fragrant.

3 Add 1 tbsp of the oil or ½ tbsp of ghee to the pan, stir through the pineapple, add the lentils and tomatoes, and a little hot water so the mixture is slightly sloppy, then simmer on a really low heat for about 15 minutes. Meanwhile, heat the remaining oil or ghee, add the prawns and cook briefly until pink, then stir them into the lentils. Taste and season if needed, stir through the coriander, and serve with rice or naan bread.

This is a mild vegetarian curry and the sweet peppers marry well with the paneer. This is an Indian cheese that won't melt upon cooking; you'll find it with the other cheeses at the supermarket.

Paneer and sweet pepper curry

 SERVES 4–6 **HEALTHY**

2 tbsp vegetable oil
1 x 230g packet paneer, cubed
10cm (4in) piece fresh root ginger, peeled and sliced
2 red chillies, deseeded and finely chopped
2 tbsp dried curry leaves, crushed
2 tsp cumin seeds

4 tsp garam masala
2 tsp ground turmeric
6 red peppers, deseeded and sliced
6 tomatoes, skinned and roughly chopped
salt and freshly ground black pepper
bunch of coriander, finely chopped

in the slow cooker   **PREP** 20 MINS   **COOK** 15 MINS PRECOOKING; AUTO/LOW 5–6 HRS OR HIGH 3–4 HRS

1 Preheat the slow cooker, if required. Heat half the oil in a heavy-based pan over a medium-high heat, add the paneer, and cook for 5–8 minutes, stirring, until golden all over. Remove and set aside.

2 Heat the remaining oil in the pan, add the ginger, chillies, curry leaves, cumin seeds, garam masala, and turmeric, and stir well to coat with the oil. Then add the peppers, tomatoes, and 100ml (3½fl oz) water and bring to the boil.

3 Transfer everything to the slow cooker, including the paneer, and season with salt and pepper. Cover with the lid and cook on auto/low for 5–6 hours or on high for 3–4 hours. Stir through the coriander and serve with rice, chapatis, or naan bread.

traditional method   **PREP** 20 MINS   **COOK** 1 HR

1 Heat half the oil in a heavy-based pan over a medium-high heat, add the paneer and cook for 5–8 minutes, stirring, until golden all over. Remove and set aside.

2 Heat the remaining oil in the pan, add the ginger, chillies, curry leaves, cumin seeds, garam masala, and turmeric, and stir well to coat with the oil. Then add the peppers and cook over a low heat for about 15 minutes until beginning to soften.

3 Add the tomatoes and 100ml (3½fl oz) water and cook on low for 15 minutes. Return the paneer to the pan, season with salt and pepper, then simmer gently for 15–20 minutes, topping up with a little hot water if needed. Stir through the coriander and serve with rice, chapatis, or naan bread.

Lots of spices enliven these red lentils, making them delicious enough to eat on their own with rice. Wash the lentils well before using and pick them over for any stones.

Red lentil dahl

◎ **SERVES** 4 ❄ **FREEZE** UP TO 3 MONTHS ♡ **HEALTHY**

1 tbsp sunflower oil
1 onion, finely chopped
salt and freshly ground black pepper
3 garlic cloves, finely chopped
1 red chilli, deseeded and finely chopped
5cm (2in) piece of fresh root ginger, peeled and grated
1 tsp ground cumin
1 tsp ground coriander
1 tsp ground turmeric

1 tsp paprika
6 curry leaves, crushed
175g (6oz) red lentils, rinsed and picked over for any stones
400g can chopped tomatoes
600ml (1 pint) hot vegetable stock for the slow cooker (900ml/1½ pints for the traditional method)
juice of ½ lemon (optional)
small bunch of coriander leaves, finely chopped

in the slow cooker   🕐 **PREP** 15 MINS   **COOK** 10 MINS PRECOOKING; AUTO/LOW 8 HRS OR **HIGH** 4 HRS

1 Preheat the slow cooker, if required. Heat the oil in a large heavy-based pan over a medium heat, add the onion, and cook for 3–4 minutes until soft. Season with salt and pepper, stir through the garlic, chilli, and ginger, and cook for a couple more minutes.

2 Add all the spices and curry leaves and stir well, then stir through the lentils so they get well coated with the spices. Tip in the tomatoes and transfer everything to the slow cooker. Pour in the stock, cover with the lid, and cook on auto/low for 8 hours or on high for 4 hours.

3 Taste and season as needed, adding the lemon juice, if using, and stir through the coriander. Serve with rice, chapatis, and a spoonful of yogurt on the side.

traditional method   🕐 **PREP** 15 MINS   **COOK** 1¼ HRS

1 Heat the oil in a large heavy-based pan over a medium heat, add the onion, and cook for 3–4 minutes until soft. Season with salt and pepper, stir through the garlic, chilli, and ginger, and cook for a couple more minutes.

2 Add all the spices and curry leaves and stir well, then stir through the lentils so they are well coated with the spices. Tip in the tomatoes and 600ml (1 pint) of the stock. Bring to the boil, then reduce to a simmer, partially cover with the lid, and cook on a low heat for about 1 hour, stirring occasionally and topping up with the reserved stock when needed.

3 Taste and season as needed, adding the lemon juice, if using, and stir through the coriander. Serve with rice, chapatis, and a spoonful of yogurt on the side.

Okra is becoming more popular, and when chopped and cooked in this way it still remains firm. Lots of ginger is the key to this dish, it works really well with the acidity of the tomatoes.

Ginger and okra curry

SERVES 4   **FREEZE** UP TO 1 MONTH   **HEALTHY**

1 tbsp sunflower oil
6 shallots, finely chopped
salt and freshly ground black pepper
1–2 green chillies, depending on your heat
   preference, deseeded and finely chopped
3 garlic cloves, finely chopped
175g (6oz) okra, tops trimmed
10cm (4in) piece of fresh root ginger, peeled
   and finely chopped

1 tsp black onion seeds
4 tomatoes, finely chopped
400g can chopped tomatoes
300ml (10fl oz) hot vegetable stock for
   the slow cooker (600ml/1 pint for the
   traditional method)
lemon wedges, for serving

in the slow cooker   PREP 15 MINS   COOK 15 MINS PRECOOKING;
AUTO/LOW 8 HRS OR HIGH 4 HRS

1 Preheat the slow cooker, if required. Heat the oil in a large heavy-based pan over a medium heat, add the shallots, and cook for about 5 minutes until soft. Season with salt and pepper, stir through the chillies and garlic, and cook for a few more minutes.

2 Add the okra, increase the heat a little and fry them, stirring, until they take on some colour. Stir in the ginger and onion seeds, turning to coat. Transfer everything to the slow cooker. Stir in the fresh and canned tomatoes and the stock. Cover with the lid and cook on auto/low for 8 hours or on high for 4 hours. Taste and season, as necessary, and serve the curry with rice, chapatis, and lemon wedges on the side.

traditional method   PREP 15 MINS   COOK 1¼ HRS

1 Heat the oil in a large heavy-based pan over a medium heat, add the shallots, and cook for about 5 minutes until soft. Season with salt and pepper, then stir through the chillies and garlic, and cook for a few more minutes.

2 Add the okra, increase the heat a little and fry them, stirring, until they take on some colour. Stir in the ginger and onion seeds, turning to coat.

3 Add the fresh and canned tomatoes and bring to the boil, then pour in the stock and let the sauce bubble for a few minutes more. Reduce to a simmer, cover with the lid, and cook on a low heat for about 1 hour, stirring occasionally and topping up with hot water if needed. For the last 15 minutes or so, remove the lid and let the sauce simmer to thicken. Taste and season, as necessary, and serve the curry with rice, chapatis, and lemon wedges on the side.

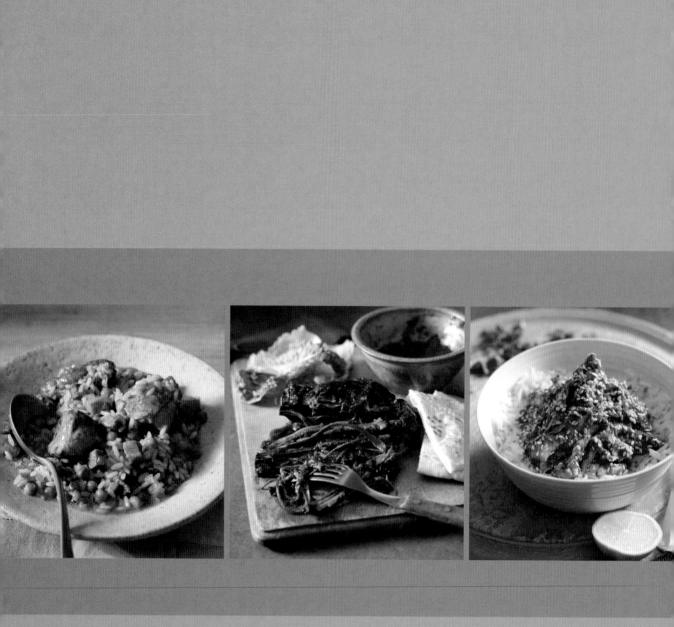

Chillies & gumbos

A blend of hot spices and dark chocolate combine in this famous Mexican dish. Turkey is a good lean meat, but use chicken if you prefer. Make sure you use the best quality dark chocolate.

Turkey mole

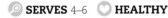 **SERVES** 4–6 **HEALTHY**

900g (2lb) boneless turkey thighs
salt and freshly ground black pepper
3 tbsp vegetable oil
45g (1½oz) dark chocolate (70 per cent cocoa),
 broken into pieces

FOR THE MOLE MIXTURE
400g can chopped tomatoes
½ onion, quartered
3 garlic cloves, peeled and left whole

1 slice of stale white bread, torn into pieces
1 stale corn tortilla, torn into pieces
175g (6oz) blanched almonds
75g (2½oz) raisins
30g (1oz) chilli powder
1 tsp each of ground cloves, coriander, and cumin
¼ tsp ground aniseed
2 tsp ground cinnamon
30g (1oz) sesame seeds

in the slow cooker   **PREP** 20 MINS   **COOK** 15 MINS PRECOOKING;
AUTO/LOW 6–8 HRS OR HIGH 3–4 HRS

1 Preheat the slow cooker, if required. Season the turkey and heat half the oil in a large flameproof casserole over a medium heat. Add the turkey pieces, skin-side down, and cook for 10–15 minutes until browned all over. Set aside. For the mole mixture, put all the ingredients, except for half the sesame seeds, in a food processor and blend to a smooth paste.

2 Heat the remaining oil in the casserole over a moderate heat, add the mole mixture, and cook, stirring, for about 5 minutes, until it is thick. Add the chocolate and stir until it has melted, then slowly add 250ml (9fl oz) of hot water, stirring. Season with salt and bring to the boil. Transfer everything to the slow cooker, including the turkey. Cover with the lid and cook on auto/low for 6–8 hours or on high for 3–4 hours. Remove the turkey and set aside until cool enough to handle. Remove the skin and any fat, and shred the meat with your fingers. Return to the sauce and stir. Taste for seasoning. Toast the remaining sesame seeds for 2–3 minutes in a dry frying pan until lightly golden. Serve with white rice and sprinkle with the sesame seeds.

traditional method   **PREP** 45–50 MINS   **COOK** 1¼–1¾ HRS

1 Season the turkey and heat half the oil in a large flameproof casserole over a medium heat. Add the turkey pieces, skin-side down, and cook for 10–15 minutes until browned all over. Add 900ml (1½ pints) water, bring to a boil, and cover. Simmer for 45–60 minutes, until the turkey is very tender when pierced with a fork. Set aside. Strain the cooking liquid into a bowl. For the mole mixture, put all the ingredients, except for half the sesame seeds, in a food processor and blend to a smooth paste.

2 Heat the remaining oil in the casserole over a moderate heat, add the mole mixture, and cook, stirring, for about 5 minutes, until it is thick. Add the chocolate and stir until it has melted. Pour in the cooking liquid, season with salt, and stir. Simmer for 25–30 minutes, to thicken. Toast the remaining sesame seeds for 2–3 minutes in a dry frying pan until lightly golden. Remove the skin and any fat from the turkey and shred the meat with your fingers. Return the turkey to the casserole and simmer for 10–15 minutes. Taste for seasoning. Serve with white rice and sprinkle with the sesame seeds.

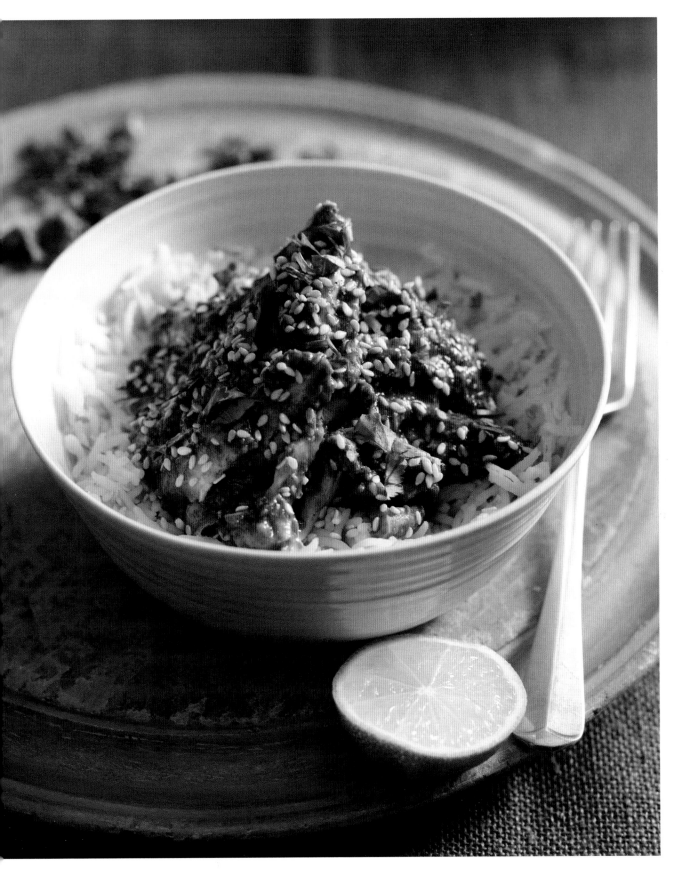

In Texas, you will never find red beans in a chilli; they are served on the side, as in this authentic recipe. Do mix them in with the meat, if you prefer. For a real Texan touch, serve it with cornbread.

Chilli con carne

SERVES 6   **FREEZE** UP TO 3 MONTHS   **HEALTHY**

3 tbsp vegetable oil, plus more if needed
1.35kg (3lb) braising steak, cut into bite-sized pieces
3 onions, chopped
3 garlic cloves, finely chopped
2 x 400g cans chopped tomatoes
2–4 dried red chillies, deseeded and finely chopped or crumbled
5–6 sprigs of fresh oregano, leaves only, or 1 tbsp dried oregano

2 tbsp chilli powder
1 tbsp paprika
2 tsp ground cumin
1–2 tsp Tabasco sauce
salt and freshly ground black pepper
1 tbsp fine cornmeal (polenta)

in the slow cooker   **PREP** 35 MINS   **COOK** 20 MINS PRECOOKING; AUTO/LOW 6–8 HRS OR **HIGH** 3–4 HRS

1 Preheat the slow cooker, if required. Heat half the oil in a large flameproof casserole over a high heat, add the beef (in batches and with extra oil, if necessary), and cook, stirring, until browned. If the meat has been cooked in batches return it all to the casserole, then add the onions, garlic, and tomatoes, and cook, stirring, for 8–10 minutes until the onions are just soft.

2 Transfer everything to the slow cooker and pour in 300ml (10fl oz) water. Stir, then add the chillies, oregano, chilli powder, paprika, cumin, Tabasco sauce, and salt and pepper. Cover with the lid and cook on auto/low for 6–8 hours or on high for 3–4 hours. Stir though the cornmeal for the last hour of cooking. At the end of cooking, the chilli should be thick and rich. Taste for seasoning, and serve it with boiled, white long-grain rice and bowls of warmed red kidney beans.

traditional method   **PREP** 35 MINS   **COOK** 2¼–2¾ HRS

1 Heat half the oil in a large flameproof casserole over a high heat, add the beef (in batches and with extra oil, if necessary), and cook, stirring, until browned. If the meat has been cooked in batches return it all to the casserole, then add the onions, garlic, and tomatoes, and cook, stirring, for 8–10 minutes until the onions are just soft.

2 Pour in 500ml (16fl oz) water and stir into the casserole with the chillies, oregano, chilli powder, paprika, cumin, Tabasco sauce, and salt and pepper. Bring just to the boil, cover, and simmer over a low heat, stirring occasionally, for about 2–2½ hours until the meat is very tender. About 30 minutes before the end of cooking, stir in the cornmeal. At the end of cooking, the chilli should be thick and rich. Taste for seasoning, and serve it with boiled, white long-grain rice and bowls of warmed red kidney beans.

In Louisiana, gumbo can be made from any number of ingredients. Best of all is prawn gumbo bolstered, as here, with oysters. It is thickened with a dark roux of flour toasted slowly in oil.

Prawn and okra gumbo

 SERVES 4–6

1 bay leaf
3–5 sprigs of thyme
1½ tsp allspice berries
1 tsp crushed chillies
75ml (2½fl oz) vegetable oil
60g (2oz) plain flour
1 large onion, finely chopped
3 garlic cloves, finely chopped
2 green peppers, deseeded and diced
salt and freshly ground black pepper
350g (12oz) tomatoes, skinned and coarsely chopped

150g (5½oz) smoked sausage, such as kielbasa, outer casing removed, if necessary, and cut into 1cm (½in) slices
250g (9oz) okra, chopped into 1cm (½in) slices
450g (1lb) raw medium prawns, peeled and deveined
12 shelled oysters
small bunch of spring onions, trimmed and sliced diagonally
small bunch of parsley, leaves finely chopped
½ tsp Tabasco sauce, plus more to taste

in the slow cooker   **PREP** 45 MINS   **COOK** 25 MINS PRECOOKING;
AUTO/LOW 6–8 HRS OR **HIGH** 3–4 HRS

1 Preheat the slow cooker, if required. Put the bay leaf, thyme, allspice, and crushed chillies in a muslin bag and tie the top. To make a roux, heat the oil in a large flameproof casserole over a low heat, stir in the flour, and cook for about 5 minutes, stirring constantly, until the roux is medium brown. Stir the onion, garlic, peppers, and seasoning into the roux and cook for 7–10 minutes, stirring, until they are softened and lightly browned. Add the tomatoes and sausage and cook, stirring occasionally, for a further 10–12 minutes. Add the okra, spice bag, and 450ml (15fl oz) water.

2 Transfer everything to the slow cooker, cover with the lid, and cook on auto/low for 6–8 hours or on high for 3–4 hours. Add the prawns for the last 10 minutes of cooking, until they start to turn pink. Add the oysters and spring onions for the last 5 minutes of cooking, until the edges of the oysters start to curl. Discard the spice bag. Stir in the parsley and Tabasco sauce. Taste for seasoning, adding more Tabasco sauce, if you like. To serve, spoon the gumbo into warmed soup bowls.

traditional method   **PREP** 45 MINS   **COOK** 1¼ HRS

1 Put the bay leaf, thyme, allspice, and crushed chillies in a muslin bag and tie the top. To make a roux, heat the oil in a large flameproof casserole over a low heat, stir in the flour, and cook for about 5 minutes, stirring constantly, until the roux is medium brown. Stir the onion, garlic, peppers, and seasoning into the roux and cook for 7–10 minutes, stirring, until they are softened and lightly browned. Add the tomatoes and sausage and cook, stirring occasionally, for a further 10–12 minutes. Add the okra, spice bag, and 450ml (15fl oz) water. Partially cover the casserole and let it simmer for 40–50 minutes until the okra is very tender and the gumbo is thick and rich.

2 Just before serving, add the prawns to the gumbo and simmer gently for 3–5 minutes until they begin to turn pink. Add the oysters and spring onions and cook for 1–2 minutes, until the edges of the oysters start to curl. Discard the spice bag. Stir in the parsley and Tabasco sauce. Taste for seasoning, adding more Tabasco sauce, if you like. To serve, spoon the gumbo into warmed soup bowls.

Pinto beans are creamy pink and, when mashed, are the common base filling of burritos. If you can't find them, use the same amount of black or kidney beans instead. They will taste just as good.

Pinto bean chilli

 SERVES 4–6 ✤ **FREEZE** UP TO 3 MONTHS ♥ **HEALTHY**

1 tbsp olive oil
2 red onions, finely chopped
salt and freshly ground black pepper
3 garlic cloves, finely chopped
2–3 red chillies, depending on your heat
  preference, deseeded and finely chopped
1 tsp ground allspice
pinch of ground cumin
1 large cinnamon stick
1 tsp dried oregano

2 bay leaves
1 tbsp cider vinegar
2 x 400g cans chopped tomatoes
1 tbsp tomato purée
1 tbsp dark brown sugar
2 x 400g cans pinto beans, drained
  and rinsed
450ml (15fl oz) hot vegetable stock
  for the slow cooker (900ml/1½ pints
  for the traditional method)

in the slow cooker 🕐 **PREP** 15 MINS **COOK** 5 MINS PRECOOKING;
                                              AUTO/LOW 6–8 HRS OR **HIGH** 4–5 HRS

1 Preheat the slow cooker, if required. Heat the oil in a large heavy-based pan over a medium heat, add the onions, and cook for 3–4 minutes until soft. Season with salt and pepper, stir in the garlic, chillies, ground spices, and herbs, and cook for 2 minutes.

2 Transfer everything to the slow cooker, then stir in the vinegar, tomatoes, tomato purée, sugar, beans, and stock. Cover with the lid and cook on auto/low for 6–8 hours or on high for 4–5 hours.

3 Taste and season as needed, removing the bay leaves and cinnamon stick, and serve with bowls of grated cheese and soured cream, if you like.

traditional method 🕐 **PREP** 15 MINS **COOK** 1½ HRS

1 Heat the oil in a large heavy-based pan over a medium heat, add the onions, and cook for 3–4 minutes until soft. Season with salt and pepper, stir in the garlic, chillies, ground spices, and herbs, and cook for 2 minutes.

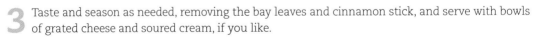

2 Add the vinegar, tomatoes, tomato purée, sugar, beans, and stock and bring to the boil. Reduce to a simmer, partially cover with the lid, and cook gently for 1–1½ hours until thickened.

3 Taste and season as needed, removing the bay leaves and cinnamon stick, and serve with bowls of grated cheese and soured cream, if you like.

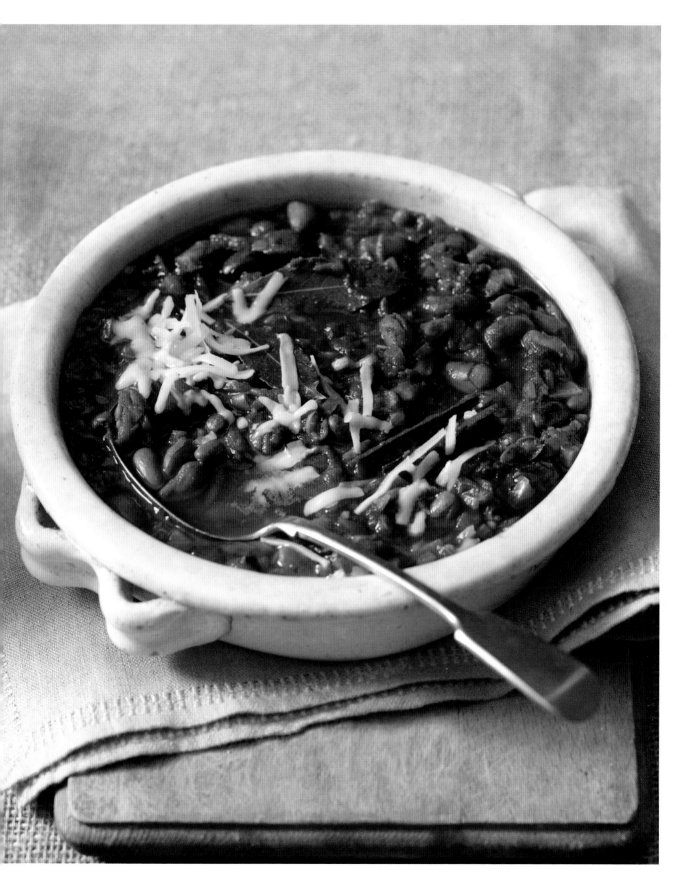

Lamb with sweet squash is the perfect combination and the minced meat benefits from long, slow cooking. Stirring mint and oregano leaves into the dish adds a distinct freshness.

Lamb mince and squash with green chillies

SERVES 4–6   **FREEZE** UP TO 1 MONTH

2 tbsp olive oil
1 butternut squash, peeled, deseeded, and chopped into bite-sized pieces
salt and freshly ground black pepper
1 onion, finely chopped
handful of fresh oregano, leaves only, or 1 tsp dried oregano
handful of thyme, leaves only
3 garlic cloves, finely chopped

1 green chilli, deseeded and finely chopped
450g (1lb) lamb mince
600ml (1 pint) hot vegetable stock for the slow cooker (900ml/1½ pints for the traditional method)
400g can chopped tomatoes
60g (2oz) sultanas
bunch of mint leaves, finely chopped
1–2 tsp harissa paste, depending on how spicy you like it

in the slow cooker   PREP 25 MINS   COOK 25 MINS PRECOOKING; AUTO/LOW 8 HRS

1 Preheat the slow cooker, if required. Heat half the oil in a large flameproof casserole over a medium heat and add the squash. Season with salt and pepper and cook for 5–8 minutes, stirring, until it starts to turn golden. Remove the squash from the casserole and set aside.

2 Heat the remaining oil in the casserole, add the onion, and cook for 3–4 minutes until soft. Stir through the oregano, thyme, garlic, and chilli, and cook for a few more minutes. Add the mince, increase the heat a little, and cook, stirring, for 5–8 minutes until it is no longer pink. Reduce the heat, return the squash to the casserole, add the stock and tomatoes, and bring to the boil. Transfer everything to the slow cooker and stir in the sultanas. Cover with the lid and cook on auto/low for 8 hours.

3 Taste and season, if necessary, then stir through the mint and harissa paste. Serve with rice or warmed pitta bread and a lightly dressed crisp green salad.

traditional method   PREP 25 MINS   COOK 1½–2 HRS

1 Preheat the oven to 180°C (350°F/Gas 4). Heat half the oil in a large flameproof casserole over a medium heat and add the squash. Season with salt and pepper and cook for 5–8 minutes, stirring, until it starts to turn golden. Remove the squash from the casserole and set aside.

2 Heat the remaining oil in the casserole, add the onion, and cook for 3–4 minutes until soft. Stir through the oregano, thyme, garlic, and chilli, and cook for a few more minutes. Add the mince, increase the heat a little, and cook, stirring, for 5–8 minutes until it is no longer pink. Reduce the heat, return the squash to the casserole, add the stock and tomatoes, and bring to the boil. Reduce to a simmer, stir through the sultanas, cover with the lid, and put in the oven for 1–1½ hours. Check occasionally that it's not drying out, topping up with a little hot water if needed.

3 Taste and season, if necessary, then stir through the mint and harissa paste. Serve with rice or warmed pitta bread and a lightly dressed crisp green salad.

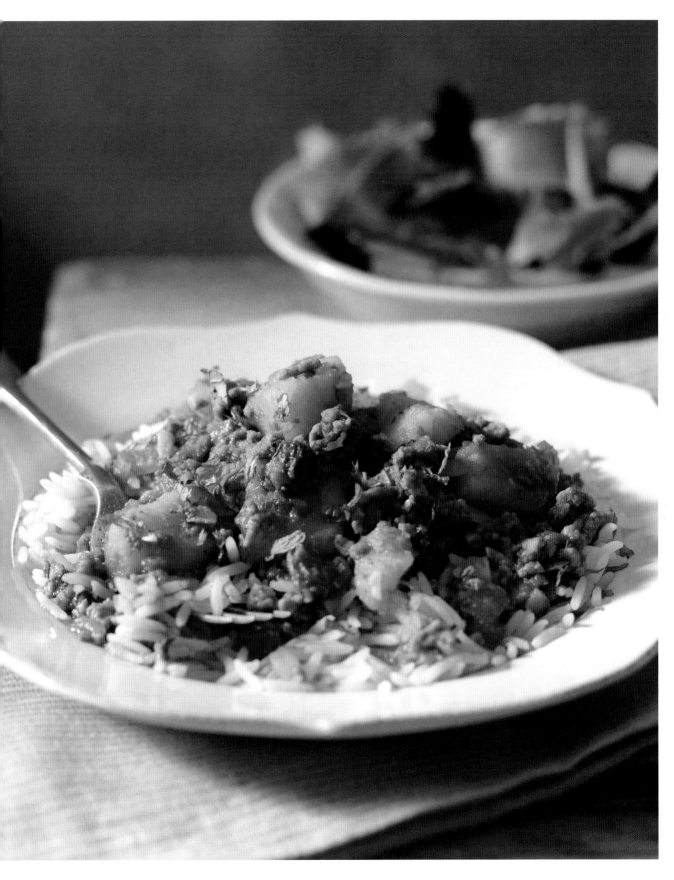

Jambalaya is a traditional southern American dish from Louisiana. Variations include spiced sausages in place of the chicken, and shrimps, which are added towards the end of the cooking time.

Chicken jambalaya

SERVES 4–6

2 tbsp olive oil
6 boneless chicken pieces (thigh and breast),
  cut into large chunky pieces
salt and freshly ground black pepper
2 tsp dried oregano
2 tsp cayenne pepper
1 red onion, finely chopped
3 garlic cloves, finely chopped
1 green pepper, deseeded and finely chopped

1 red pepper, deseeded and finely chopped
200g (7oz) thick slices ready-cooked ham,
  roughly chopped
600ml (1 pint) hot chicken stock for the slow
  cooker (900ml/1½ pints for the traditional
  method), plus extra if necessary
175g (6oz) easy-cook long-grain rice
140g (5oz) frozen or fresh peas
small handful of coriander, finely chopped (optional)

in the slow cooker   **PREP** 15–20 MINS   **COOK** 20 MINS PRECOOKING; AUTO/LOW 2–3 HRS

1 Preheat the slow cooker, if required. Heat half the oil in a large flameproof casserole over a medium-high heat. Season the chicken pieces with salt and pepper, toss in the oregano and cayenne pepper, then add to the casserole (in batches, if necessary) and cook for 6–10 minutes until golden brown. Remove and set aside.

2 Heat the remaining oil in the casserole over a medium heat, add the onion, garlic, and peppers, and cook for 5–8 minutes, stirring. Transfer everything to the slow cooker, including the chicken. Add the ham and pour in enough stock to just cover the meat. Stir in the rice and peas, then season, cover with the lid, and cook on auto/low for 2–3 hours or until all the liquid has been absorbed, stirring after an hour of cooking.

3 Taste and add seasoning, if needed, and stir in the coriander, if using. Try serving with a green salad, green beans, plain yogurt or soured cream, and some crusty bread.

traditional method   **PREP** 15–20 MINS   **COOK** 1½ HRS

1 Heat half the oil in a large flameproof casserole over a medium-high heat. Season the chicken pieces with salt and pepper, toss in the oregano and cayenne pepper, then add to the casserole (in batches, if necessary) and cook for 6–10 minutes until golden brown. Remove and set aside.

2 Heat the remaining oil in the casserole over a medium heat, add the onion, garlic, and peppers and cook for 5–8 minutes, stirring. Return the chicken to the casserole and stir in the ham. Pour in the stock and bring to the boil, then reduce to a simmer, season well, partially cover with the lid, and cook gently for about 40 minutes. Check occasionally that it's not drying out, topping up with a little hot water if needed. Stir in the rice, turning so it absorbs all the stock, and cook for about 15 minutes or until the rice is cooked, topping up with more stock, if necessary. Add the peas for the last 5 minutes.

3 Taste and add seasoning, if needed, and stir in the coriander, if using. Try serving with a green salad, green beans, plain yogurt or soured cream, and some crusty bread.

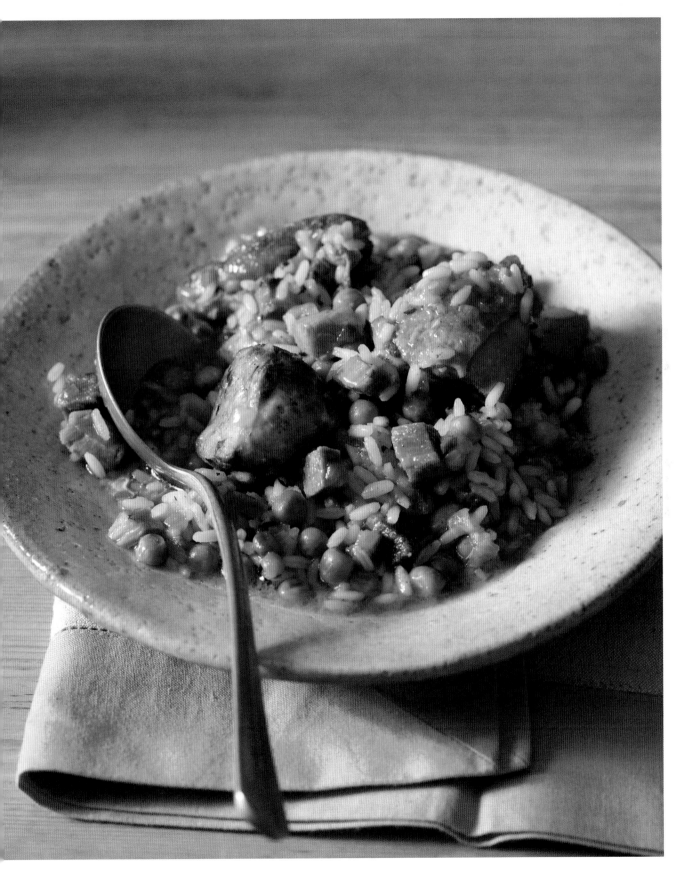

The black beans in this recipe become fabulously tender when cooked in the coconut milk. Add lots of chilli and garlic and the result is a tasty vegetarian dish.

Spicy black beans and coconut

SERVES 4–6

175g (6oz) black beans, soaked overnight
  and drained
1 tbsp olive oil
1 onion, very finely chopped
salt and freshly ground black pepper

5 garlic cloves, finely chopped
2 red chillies, deseeded and finely chopped
2 x 400ml cans coconut milk
450ml (15fl oz) hot vegetable stock, for
  both methods

in the slow cooker   **PREP** 10 MINS, PLUS SOAKING   **COOK** 20 MINS PRECOOKING; AUTO/LOW 8 HRS

1 Preheat the slow cooker, if required. Put the black beans in a large heavy-based pan and cover with plenty of water. Bring to the boil, cover with the lid, and cook for 10 minutes. Drain and set the beans aside in a bowl. Heat the oil in the pan over a medium heat, add the onion, and cook for 3–4 minutes until soft. Season with salt and pepper, then stir in the garlic and chilli. Return the beans to the pan and turn until well coated.

2 Tip in the coconut milk and stock, season again, and bring the sauce to the boil. Transfer everything to the slow cooker, cover with the lid, and cook on auto/low for 8 hours. Taste and season as required and serve with warm bowls of rice.

traditional method   **PREP** 10 MINS, PLUS SOAKING   **COOK** 1¾–2¼ HRS

1 Preheat the oven to 160°C (325°F/Gas 3). Put the black beans in a large heavy-based pan and cover with plenty of water. Bring to the boil, cover with the lid, and cook for 10 minutes. Drain and set the beans aside in a bowl. Heat the oil in the pan over a medium heat, add the onion, and cook for 3–4 minutes until soft. Season with salt and pepper, then stir in the garlic and chilli. Return the beans to the pan and turn until well coated.

2 Tip in the coconut milk and stock, season again, and bring the sauce to the boil. Cover with the lid and put in the oven for 1½–2 hours or until the beans are soft. Check occasionally that it's not drying out, topping up with a little hot water if needed. Taste and season as required and serve with warm bowls of rice.

This highly flavoured, gutsy dish is guaranteed to make the taste buds tingle. To make the most of its flavours, enjoy the jambalaya on its own with a simple salad and crusty bread.

Sausage and shrimp jambalaya

SERVES 6　　**FREEZE** UP TO 3 MONTHS

1–2 tbsp olive oil
250g (9oz) smoked sausage, cut into bite-sized pieces
250g (9oz) chorizo, chopped into thick slices
2 onions, diced
1 green pepper, deseeded and diced
1 red pepper, deseeded and diced
salt and freshly ground black pepper
3 garlic cloves, peeled and finely chopped
2 tsp Cajun seasoning

1 tbsp plain flour
about 450ml (15fl oz) hot chicken stock for the slow cooker (900ml/1½ pints for the traditional method)
2 tbsp Worcestershire sauce
300g (10oz) easy-cook rice
2 bay leaves
250g (9oz) shrimps or small prawns
250g (9oz) okra, sliced
handful of flat-leaf parsley, finely chopped

in the slow cooker　　**PREP** 15 MINS　**COOK** 15 MINS PRECOOKING; AUTO/LOW 3–4 HRS OR HIGH 1–2 HRS

1 Preheat the slow cooker, if required. Heat the oil in a large flameproof casserole over a medium-high heat, add the sausage and chorizo, and cook for 5–8 minutes until golden. Remove and set aside.

2 Reduce the heat to medium, add the onions, and cook for 3–4 minutes until soft. Stir through the peppers and cook for a few more minutes, until beginning to soften. Add seasoning, stir though the garlic and Cajun seasoning, and cook for 1 minute. Stir through the flour to combine and ladle in a little stock. Return the sausages and chorizo and add the Worcestershire sauce.

3 Transfer everything to the slow cooker, stir through the rice and bay leaves, then pour over just enough stock to cover. Cover with the lid and cook on auto/low for 3–4 hours or on high for 1–2 hours. Add the shrimps or prawns and okra for the last hour of cooking. Remove the bay leaves, taste and season if needed, then stir through the parsley. Serve with a salad and some crusty bread.

traditional method　　**PREP** 15 MINS　**COOK** 2¼ HRS

1 Preheat the oven to 150°C (300°F/Gas 2). Heat the oil in a large flameproof casserole over a medium-high heat, add the sausage and chorizo, and cook for 5–8 minutes until golden. Remove and set aside.

2 Reduce the heat to medium, add the onions, and cook for 3–4 minutes until soft. Stir through the pepper and cook for a few more minutes, until beginning to soften. Add seasoning, stir though the garlic and Cajun seasoning, and cook for 1 minute. Stir through the flour to combine and ladle in a little stock. Return the sausages, chorizo, and peppers and add the Worcestershire sauce.

3 Stir through the rice and bay leaves, then pour over the stock. Mix well, cover with the lid, and put in the oven for 1½ hours. Check occasionally that it's not drying out, topping up with a little hot water if needed. Stir in the shrimps or prawns and okra, re-cover, and cook for a further 30 minutes. Remove the bay leaves, taste and season if needed, then stir through the parsley. Serve with a salad and some crusty bread.

The basis of this tasty stew is sweetcorn. If you can't get hold of creamed sweetcorn, use a can of regular sweetcorn and blend it in the food processor. Omit the fish if you are cooking for vegetarians.

Creole fish and corn stew

⚙ **SERVES** 4–6　❄ **FREEZE** UP TO 1 MONTH　♡ **HEALTHY**

2 tbsp olive oil
1 onion, finely chopped
3 garlic cloves, finely chopped
3 celery sticks, finely chopped
3 carrots, peeled and finely chopped
1 tsp dried oregano
few sprigs of thyme, leaves only
1 tsp cayenne pepper (use less if you
　don't like it too hot)
400g can creamed sweetcorn

400g can sweetcorn, drained
600ml (1 pint) hot vegetable stock for the slow
　cooker (900ml/1½ pints for the traditional method)
salt and freshly ground black pepper
2 potatoes, peeled and diced into bite-sized pieces
200g (7oz) ready-cooked prawns, chopped
300g (10oz) white fish, skinned and cut into
　chunky pieces
splash of Tabasco sauce (optional)

in the slow cooker　🕐 **PREP** 15 MINS　**COOK** 10 MINS PRECOOKING; **HIGH** 3–4 HRS

1 Preheat the slow cooker, if required. Heat the oil in a large heavy-based pan over a medium heat, add the onion, and cook for 3–4 minutes until soft. Then stir through the garlic, celery, and carrot, and cook on a gentle heat for a further 5 minutes, or until the carrot is soft.

2 Stir through the herbs and cayenne pepper, then add both the cans of sweetcorn. Transfer everything to the slow cooker, pour in the stock, season with salt and pepper, and then add the potatoes.

3 Cover with the lid and cook on high for 3–4 hours. For the last 15 minutes of cooking, add the prawns and fish and cook until the fish is opaque and cooked through. Taste and season further, if necessary, and stir in the Tabasco sauce, if using. Ladle into warmed bowls and serve with crusty bread.

traditional method　🕐 **PREP** 15 MINS　**COOK** 1¼ HRS

1 Heat the oil in a large heavy-based pan over a medium heat, add the onion, and cook for 3–4 minutes until soft. Then stir through the garlic, celery, and carrot, and cook on a gentle heat for a further 5 minutes or until the carrot is soft.

2 Stir through the herbs and cayenne pepper, then add both the cans of sweetcorn and the stock. Season well with salt and pepper, bring to the boil, reduce to a simmer and cook gently, partially covered, for 30–40 minutes. Add the potatoes and cook for a further 15 minutes.

3 Add the prawns and fish to the casserole and simmer gently for 6–10 minutes, until the fish is opaque and cooked through. Taste and season further, if necessary, and stir in the Tabasco sauce, if using. Ladle into warmed bowls and serve with crusty bread.

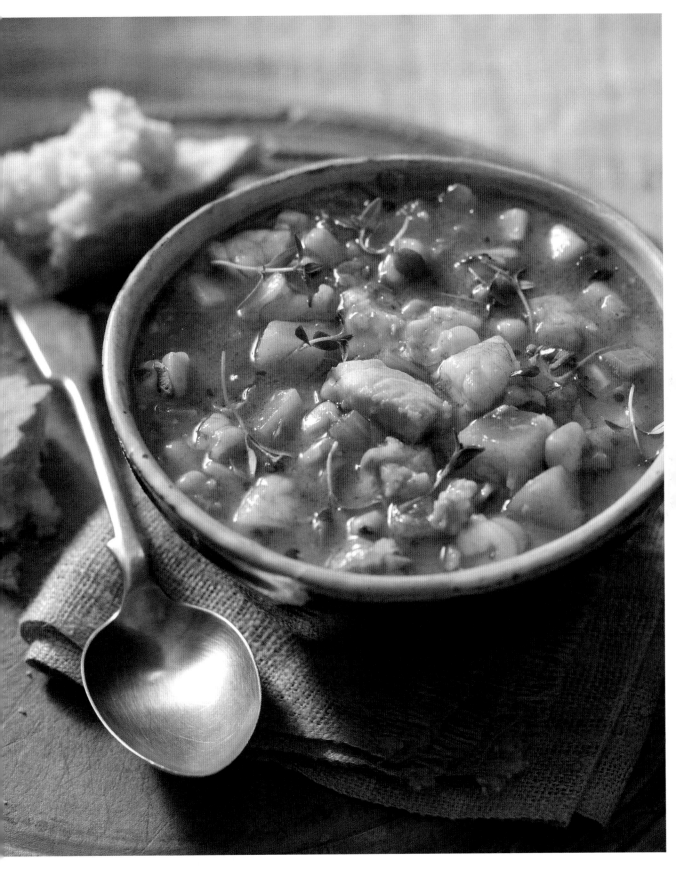

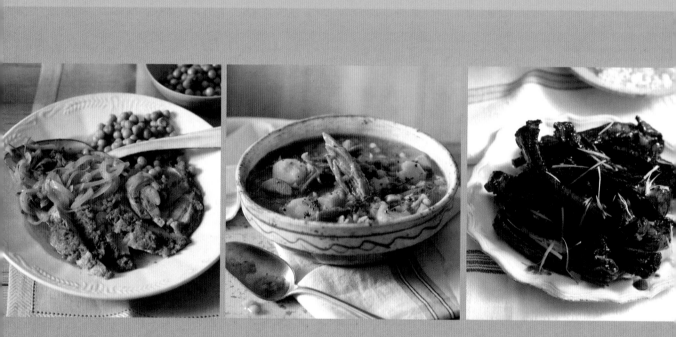

Pot roasts & ribs

This beef is slow cooked in sweet Madeira for maximum flavour. Buy the meat in one piece from your butcher and don't forget to soak the dried porcini mushrooms in water for 20 minutes.

Beef pot roast

⊘ SERVES 4–6   **❄ FREEZE** UP TO 1 MONTH

2 tbsp olive oil
900g (2lb) whole piece of chuck beef
salt and freshly ground black pepper
1 large onion, chopped into eighths
1 tbsp wholegrain mustard
150ml (5fl oz) Madeira wine

30g (1oz) dried porcini mushrooms, soaked in 120ml (4fl oz) warm water for 20 mins, strained, and liquid reserved
600ml (1 pint) hot beef stock for the slow cooker (900ml/1½ pints for the traditional method)
handful of flat-leaf parsley, finely chopped

in the slow cooker   ⏱ **PREP** 10 MINS, PLUS SOAKING   **COOK** 25 MINS PRECOOKING; AUTO/LOW 8 HRS

1 Preheat the slow cooker, if required. Heat half the oil in a large flameproof casserole over a medium-high heat. Season the beef with salt and pepper, add it to the casserole, and cook for 6–8 minutes on each side until golden. It is ready when it lifts away from the bottom of the casserole easily. Remove and set aside.

2 Heat the remaining oil in the casserole over a medium heat, add the onion, and cook for 3–4 minutes until soft. Stir through the mustard, increase the heat, and add the Madeira wine. Cook for a minute, then add the drained mushrooms.

3 Transfer everything to the slow cooker, including the beef. Add the stock and about 100ml (3½fl oz) of the strained mushroom liquid. Cover with the lid and cook on auto/low for 8 hours. Taste and season as necessary. Sprinkle with parsley and serve with mashed potatoes or baby cubed roast potatoes.

traditional method   ⏱ **PREP** 10 MINS, PLUS SOAKING   **COOK** 2½ HRS

1 Preheat the oven to 160°C (325°F/Gas 3). Heat half the oil in a large flameproof casserole over a medium-high heat. Season the beef with salt and pepper, add it to the casserole, and cook for 6–8 minutes on each side until golden. It is ready when it lifts away from the bottom of the casserole easily. Remove and set aside.

2 Heat the remaining oil in the casserole over a medium heat, add the onion, and cook for 3–4 minutes until soft. Stir through the mustard, increase the heat, and add the Madeira wine. Cook for a minute, then add the drained mushrooms, beef stock, and about 100ml (3½fl oz) of the strained mushroom liquid. Bring to the boil and stir, then reduce to a simmer and return the beef to the casserole.

3 Cover with the lid and put in the oven for 2 hours. Check occasionally that it's not drying out, topping up with a little hot water if needed. Be careful not to add too much, however, or this will dilute the flavour. Taste and season as necessary. Sprinkle with parsley and serve with mashed potatoes or baby cubed roast potatoes.

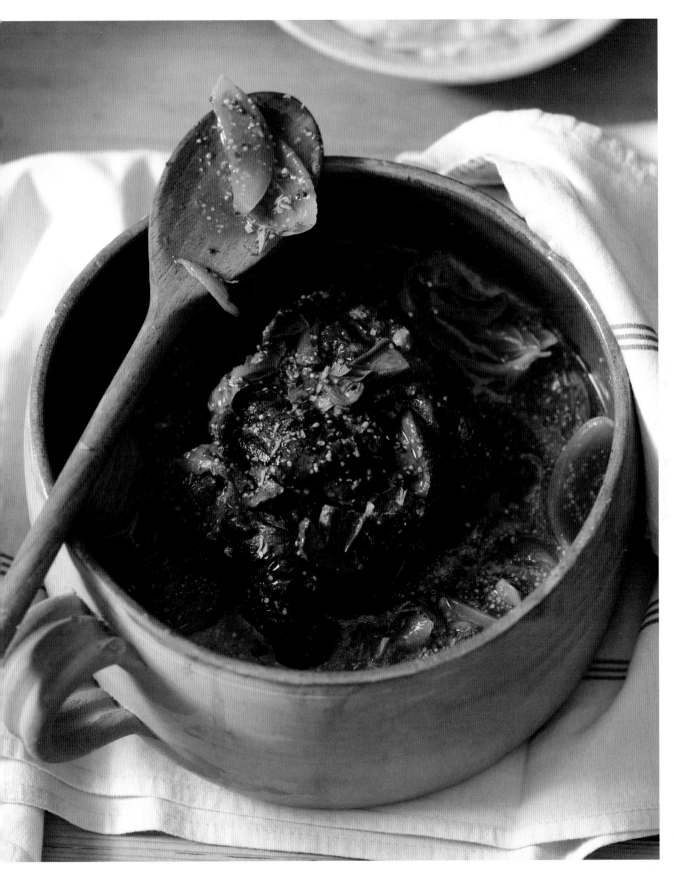

Chicken wings are cheap to buy and have lots of succulent meat on them. Serve these moreish, sticky charred chicken wings with a fiery hot dip or with something cool, such as a blue cheese dip.

Buffalo chicken wings

SERVES 4

2 tbsp olive oil, plus extra for oiling
1 shallot, finely chopped
1 garlic clove, crushed
2 tbsp tomato purée
1 tbsp dried oregano

few drops of Tabasco sauce
2 tsp light soft brown sugar
salt and freshly ground black pepper
12 chicken wings, tips removed

in the slow cooker   PREP 20 MINS, PLUS MARINATING   COOK AUTO/LOW 5–6 HRS

1 Preheat the slow cooker, if required. Place the oil, shallot, garlic, tomato purée, oregano, Tabasco, and sugar in a food processor, season with salt and pepper, and blend to a paste. Spoon into a large food bag and add the chicken wings. Shake the bag until the meat is well coated with the marinade, then chill in the refrigerator for at least 30 minutes to marinate.

2 Put the chicken wings and marinade into the slow cooker, spreading them evenly across the bottom. Cover with the lid and cook on auto/low for 5–6 hours, turning them halfway through the cooking time, if you wish. Serve with a spicy chilli, tomato, and coriander dip or a blue cheese dip and some salad.

traditional method   PREP 20 MINS, PLUS MARINATING   COOK 40 MINS

1 Place the oil, shallot, garlic, tomato purée, oregano, Tabasco, and sugar in a food processor, season with salt and pepper, and blend to a paste. Spoon into a large food bag and add the chicken wings. Shake the bag until the meat is well coated with the marinade, then chill in the refrigerator for at least 30 minutes to marinate.

2 Preheat the oven to 160°C (325°F/Gas 3). Remove the chicken wings from the bag and lay them, skin-side down, on 2 lightly oiled baking trays. Put in the oven for 20 minutes. Turn the chicken wings over and cook for a further 20 minutes or until cooked through. Serve with a spicy chilli, tomato, and coriander dip or a blue cheese dip and some salad.

Gherkins, sea salt, and mustard are the classic accompaniments to a pot au feu. It can be served as two courses – first, the rich cooking broth, then the meat and vegetables to follow.

Pot au feu

SERVES 4–6

1kg (2¼lb) boneless beef shin, tied with string lengthways at 2.5cm (1in) intervals
675g (1½lb) beef blade steak
600ml (1 pint) hot chicken stock for the slow cooker (4 litres/7 pints for the traditional method)
1 onion, peeled and studded with 2 cloves
1 large bouquet garni, made with 12–15 sprigs of parsley, 4–5 sprigs of thyme, and 2 bay leaves
salt

10 peppercorns
500g (1lb 2oz) carrots, chopped into 7.5cm (3in) lengths
1 small head of celery, chopped into 7.5cm (3in) lengths
350g (12oz) leeks, chopped into 7.5cm (3in) lengths
about 1kg (2¼lb) marrow bones (optional)
½ French loaf, sliced diagonally and toasted

in the slow cooker ⏱ **PREP** 40 MINS **COOK** 10 MINS PRECOOKING; **AUTO/LOW** 6–8 HRS

1 Preheat the slow cooker, if required. Put the shin, blade steak, and stock in the slow cooker and add the onion, bouquet garni, a pinch of salt, and the peppercorns. Cover with the lid and cook on auto/low for 6–8 hours. Tie the carrots, celery, leeks, and marrow bones, if using, each in a separate bundle of muslin and add to the slow cooker for the last 2 hours of cooking, along with salt for seasoning.

2 Remove the meat and marrow bones from the broth. Discard the strings from the beef shin and cut it into slices, then cut the blade steak into pieces, discarding any bones. Remove the vegetable bundles, unwrap, and arrange them on a serving platter with the meat. Cover with foil and keep warm.

3 Strain the broth into a clean pan and taste for seasoning. If necessary, boil it until reduced and well flavoured. If using the marrow bones, scoop out the marrow with a teaspoon and spread it on the slices of toast. Discard the bones. Place the toast in warmed bowls, pour over the hot broth, and serve immediately with the meat and vegetables.

traditional method ⏱ **PREP** 40 MINS **COOK** 3½–4 HRS

1 Put the shin, blade steak, and stock in a large flameproof casserole. Bring to the boil, skimming. Add the onion, bouquet garni, a pinch of salt, and the peppercorns. Simmer gently, uncovered, for 2 hours, skimming occasionally. Tie the carrots, celery, leeks, and marrow bones, if using, each in a separate bundle of muslin and add to the casserole. Season with salt. Simmer for 1½–2 hours until the meat and vegetables are very tender. Add more hot water if needed to ensure everything is always covered.

2 Remove the meat and marrow bones from the broth. Discard the strings from the beef shin and cut it into slices, then cut the blade steak into pieces, discarding any bones. Remove the vegetable bundles, unwrap, and arrange them on a serving platter with the meat. Cover with foil and keep warm.

3 Strain the broth into a clean pan and taste for seasoning. If necessary, boil it until reduced and well flavoured. If using the marrow bones, scoop out the marrow with a teaspoon and spread it on the slices of toast. Discard the bones. Place the toast in warmed bowls, pour over the hot broth, and serve immediately with the meat and vegetables.

Knuckle or ham hock is amazing value, and tasty, too.
The Jerusulem artichokes add a nutty, creamy texture,
but if they're not available you can use parsnips instead.

Pot roast smoked ham

⊚ **SERVES** 4–6 ✹ **FREEZE** UP TO 1 MONTH

2 smoked ham hocks (knuckles), about
  1.35kg (3lb) each
1 bay leaf
1 tbsp olive oil
1 onion, finely chopped
salt and freshly ground black pepper
3 garlic cloves, finely chopped

few sprigs of thyme
3 carrots, peeled and chopped
225g (8oz) Jerusalem artichokes, peeled and sliced
125g (4½oz) yellow split peas
100ml (3½fl oz) dry cider
600ml (1 pint) hot vegetable stock for the slow
  cooker (900ml/1½ pints for the traditional method)

in the slow cooker 🕑 **PREP** 25 MINS **COOK** 15 MINS PRECOOKING; **AUTO/LOW** 8 HRS OR
                        HIGH 4 HRS, THEN **AUTO/LOW** 8 HRS OR **HIGH** 4 HRS

1 Preheat the slow cooker, if required. Put the ham hocks and bay leaf in the slow cooker and pour over 1.7 litres (3 pints) of water. Cook on auto/low for 8 hours or on high for 4 hours. Remove the hams and, when cool enough to handle, peel away the skins and discard. Set the hams aside. (You can reserve the stock and use it if you wish, but it can be salty.)

2 Heat the oil in a large heavy-based pan over a medium heat, add the onion, and cook for 3–4 minutes until soft. Season with salt and pepper, stir through the garlic, thyme, carrots, and artichokes, and cook for a few more minutes. Stir through the split peas to coat. Increase the heat and pour in the cider, let it bubble for a minute, then add the stock. Transfer everything to the slow cooker, including the hams, tucking them down as much as possible. Cover with the lid and cook on auto/low for 8 hours or on high for 4 hours. The ham meat should now slide off the bone, so remove it with a fork and stir into the slow cooker. Taste and season, if necessary, and serve with some crusty bread.

traditional method 🕑 **PREP** 25 MINS **COOK** 3¼ HRS

1 Put the ham hocks and bay leaf in a large heavy-based pan, cover with water, and cook for about 2 hours, skimming away any scum that comes to the top of the pan. Remove the hams and, when cool enough to handle, peel away the skins and discard. Set the hams aside. (You can reserve the stock and use it if you wish, but it can be salty.)

2 Preheat the oven to 180°C (350°F/Gas 4). Heat the oil in a large flameproof casserole over a medium heat, add the onion, and cook for 3–4 minutes until soft. Season with salt and pepper, stir through the garlic, thyme, carrots, and artichokes, and cook for a few more minutes. Stir through the split peas to coat. Increase the heat and pour in the cider, let it bubble for a minute, then add the stock and bring to the boil. Reduce to a simmer and return the hams, tucking them down as much as possible.

3 Cover and put in the oven for about 1 hour or until the split peas are soft. Check occasionally that it's not drying out too much, topping up with hot water if needed. The ham meat should now slide off the bone, so remove it with a fork and stir into the casserole. Taste and season, if necessary, and serve with some crusty bread.

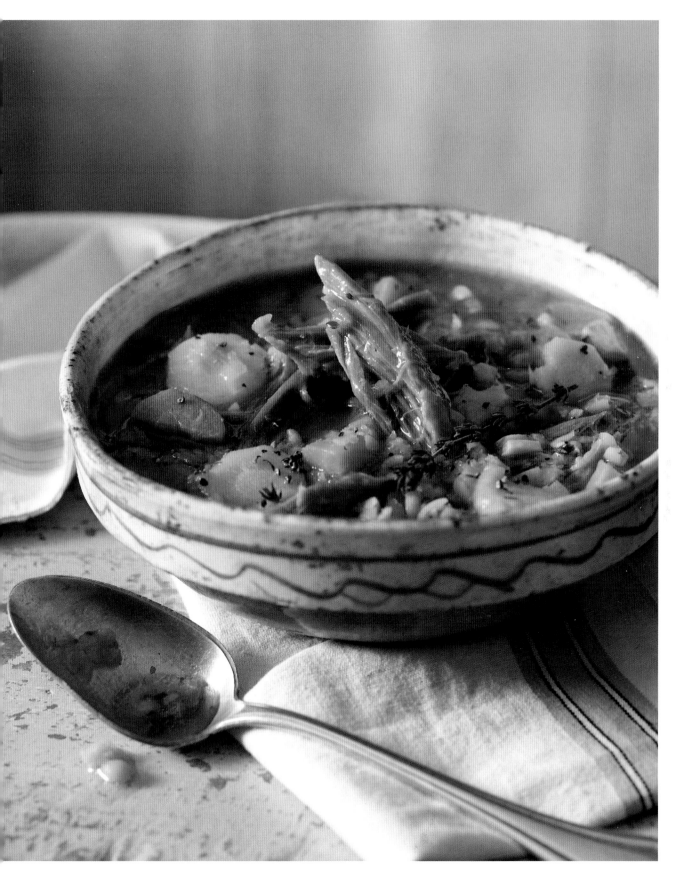

Pot roasting a pheasant retains all its flavour and moistness. Choose a plump bird meaty enough for four. Otherwise, if your slow cooker will accommodate it, use two pheasants.

Pot roast pheasant

SERVES 4

2 tbsp olive oil
60g (2oz) butter, chilled
1 prepared pheasant, about 1kg (2¼lb)
salt and freshly ground black pepper
250g (9oz) chestnut mushrooms

2 tbsp chopped thyme
1 large onion, finely chopped
100g (3½oz) rindless streaky bacon, chopped
750ml (1¼ pints) red wine, for both methods

in the slow cooker   **PREP** 40 MINS   **COOK** 20 MINS PRECOOKING; **AUTO/LOW** 6–8 HRS

1 Preheat the slow cooker, if required. Heat half the oil and half the butter in a large flameproof casserole. Brown the pheasant evenly for 6–8 minutes and season with salt and pepper. Remove and set aside. Add the mushrooms and thyme to the casserole and cook for 5 minutes, or until coloured. Also remove and set aside.

2 Heat the remaining oil in the casserole, add the onion and bacon, and cook for 4–5 minutes until the onion softens. Transfer to the slow cooker, together with the pheasant and mushrooms, and add the wine. Cover with the lid and cook on auto/low for 6–8 hours. Remove the pheasant to a serving platter, cover with foil, and keep warm.

3 Strain the liquid from the slow cooker into a heavy-based pan. Skim away any fat, then bring to the boil and simmer briskly for about 10 minutes until reduced by a third. Whisk in the remaining butter to make the sauce glossy. Carve the pheasant and serve with the hot gravy and some carrots, swede mash, and French beans.

traditional method   **PREP** 40 MINS   **COOK** 1¾ HRS

1 Preheat the oven to 190°C (375°F/Gas 5). Heat half the oil and half the butter in a large flameproof casserole. Brown the pheasant evenly for 6–8 minutes and season with salt and pepper. Remove and set aside. Add the mushrooms and thyme to the casserole and cook for 5 minutes or until coloured. Also remove and set aside.

2 Heat the remaining oil in the casserole, add the onion and bacon, and cook for 4–5 minutes until the onion softens. Add the pheasant and mushrooms and then the wine. Cover and put in the oven for 1½ hours, or until the pheasant is cooked and a leg pulls away from the bird easily. Remove the pheasant to a serving platter, cover with foil, and keep warm.

3 Strain the liquid from the casserole into a heavy-based pan. Skim away any fat, then bring to the boil and simmer briskly for about 10 minutes until reduced by a third. Whisk in the remaining butter to make the sauce glossy. Carve the pheasant and serve with the hot gravy and some carrots, swede mash, and French beans.

Slow cooking is the best way to transform brisket into tender, succulent meat that just falls into the sauce. The red onion adds a sweetness to balance the bitter Guiness in this dish.

Beef brisket and baby onions

SERVES 4–6

1 tbsp olive oil
1.1kg (2½lb) beef brisket
salt and freshly ground black pepper
2 red onions, roughly chopped
12 baby onions, peeled and left whole
2 celery sticks, roughly chopped
3 garlic cloves, finely chopped

1 bay leaf
6 juniper berries
200ml (7fl oz) Guinness
450ml (15fl oz) hot beef stock for the slow cooker
  (900ml/1½ pints for the traditional method)
3 carrots, peeled and roughly sliced
2 sprigs of rosemary

in the slow cooker   **PREP** 20 MINS   **COOK** 15 MINS PRECOOKING; **AUTO/LOW** 8 HRS

1 Preheat the slow cooker, if required. Heat the oil in a large flameproof casserole over a medium-high heat, season the brisket with salt and pepper, and add to the casserole. Cook for 6–8 minutes on each side, using tongs to turn it. It is ready when it comes away from the bottom of the pan easily. Remove from the casserole and set aside.

2 Add the red onions to the casserole and cook in the meat fat for about 10 minutes until they begin to soften. Add seasoning, then stir in the baby onions, pushing the red ones to one side a little so they get some colour. Cook for about 5 minutes, then add the celery and garlic, bay leaf, and juniper berries and cook for a further 5 minutes.

3 Pour in the Guinness and a little stock, and bring to the boil. Then add the carrots, rosemary, and the remaining stock and bring to the boil. Transfer everything to the slow cooker, including the brisket, cover with the lid, and cook on auto/low for 8 hours. To serve, slice or shred the brisket and spoon over the juices and vegetables, removing the rosemary stalks. Serve with mashed potatoes.

traditional method   **PREP** 20 MINS   **COOK** 2–2½ HRS

1 Preheat the oven to 180°C (350°F/Gas 4). Heat the oil in a large flameproof casserole over a medium-high heat, season the brisket with salt and pepper, and add to the casserole. Cook for 6–8 minutes on each side, using tongs to turn it. It is ready when it comes away from the bottom of the casserole easily. Remove and set aside.

2 Add the red onions to the casserole and cook in the meat fat for about 10 minutes until they begin to soften. Add seasoning, then stir in the baby onions, pushing the red ones to one side a little so they get some colour. Cook for about 5 minutes, then add the celery and garlic, bay leaf, and juniper berries and cook for a further 5 minutes.

3 Pour in the Guinness and a little stock, increase the heat, and let it bubble for few minutes. Then add the carrots, rosemary, and the remaining stock and bring to the boil. Reduce to a simmer, return the brisket to the casserole, cover with the lid, and put in the oven for 1½–2 hours. Spoon over the juices halfway through to keep it moist. To serve, slice or shred the brisket and spoon over the juices and vegetables, removing the rosemary stalks. Serve with mashed potatoes.

Rather than using ground pepper to season the ribs, use black peppercorns to give it more of a spicy hit. The marinade cooks to a lovely, thick, sticky coating – you'll need napkins to hand.

Spicy devilled pork ribs

SERVES 4

rack of pork ribs, about 12 ribs
   (about 700g/1lb 9oz)
salt
2 tsp black peppercorns

FOR THE MARINADE
2 tbsp tomato ketchup
1 tbsp English mustard
1 tbsp Worcestershire sauce
3 garlic cloves, finely chopped
2 tbsp runny honey
2 tbsp soy sauce
splash of smoked Tabasco sauce
small bunch of coriander, very finely chopped

in the slow cooker   **PREP** 5 MINS   **COOK** AUTO/LOW 6–8 HRS

1 Preheat the slow cooker, if required. Chop the rack into ribs and put in the slow cooker. Season with salt and add the peppercorns. Mix all the marinade ingredients together in a bowl, add to the slow cooker, and turn the ribs to coat. Cover with the lid and cook on auto/low for 6–8 hours, turning them halfway through the cooking time. Remove from the slow cooker and serve while piping hot.

traditional method   **PREP** 5 MINS   **COOK** 2–2½ HRS

1 Put the rack of ribs in a large heavy-based pan and cover with water. Season with salt and add the peppercorns. Bring to the boil, then reduce to a simmer, partially cover with the lid, and cook for 1–1½ hours until the meat starts to come away from the bone. Remove from the pan and set aside until cool enough to handle.

2 Preheat the oven to 160°C (325°F/Gas 3). Mix all the marinade ingredients together in a bowl. Chop the rack into ribs, then sit them in a large flameproof casserole. Pour over the marinade and turn the ribs to coat. Cover with the lid and put in the oven for about 1 hour, keeping an eye on them so they don't dry out; they may need turning in the marinade to prevent this from happening. Remove from the casserole and serve while piping hot.

Shanks are ideal for slow cooking as the meat melts off the bone into the sauce to create the most gorgeous tasting dish. Tart vinegar and tomato purée counteract the fattiness of the lamb.

Sweet and sour lamb

SERVES 4–6

4–6 lamb shanks (allow 1 per person)
salt and freshly ground black pepper
1–2 tbsp olive oil
1 onion, cut into eighths
2 tbsp tomato purée
4 tbsp red wine vinegar

2 tbsp demerara brown sugar
300ml (½ pint) hot vegetable stock for the slow cooker (450ml/15fl oz for the traditional method)
1 cinnamon stick
1 Savoy cabbage or dark green cabbage, trimmed and shredded

in the slow cooker   **PREP** 15 MINS   **COOK** 20 MINS PRECOOKING; AUTO/LOW 6–8 HRS

1 Preheat the slow cooker, if required. Season the lamb with salt and pepper. Heat the oil in a large flameproof casserole over a medium-high heat, add the meat, and cook (in batches, if necessary) for 10–15 minutes, turning several times, until browned all over. Reduce the heat to medium, add the onion, and cook for 3–4 minutes until soft.

2 Add the tomato purée, vinegar, and sugar and pour over 300ml (10fl oz) of water. Bring to the boil, then transfer everything to the slow cooker. Add the stock and cinnamon stick, cover with the lid, and cook on auto/low for 6–8 hours. Add the cabbage for the last 30 minutes of cooking. Taste and season as required and serve on a bed of fluffy rice.

traditional method   **PREP** 15 MINS   **COOK** 2 HRS

1 Preheat the oven to 160°C (325°F/Gas 3). Season the lamb with salt and pepper. Heat the oil in a large flameproof casserole over a medium-high heat, add the meat, and cook (in batches, if necessary) for 10–15 minutes, turning several times, until browned all over. Reduce the heat to medium, add the onion, and cook for 3–4 minutes until soft.

2 Add the tomato purée, vinegar, and sugar and pour over 300ml (10fl oz) of water. Bring to the boil, then add the stock and cinnamon stick, cover with the lid, and put in the oven for about 1½ hours. Check occasionally that it's not drying out, topping up with a little hot water if needed. Add the cabbage for the last 20 minutes of cooking. Taste and season as required and serve on a bed of fluffy rice.

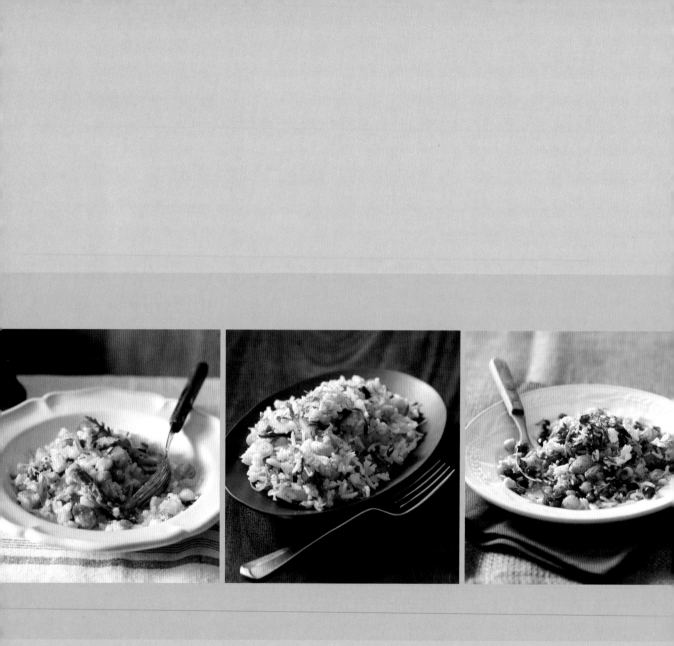

Risottos, pilafs, & paellas

Full of spring flavours – you can mix and match vegetables, such as French beans or broccoli, depending on what you have to hand. You could use chicken stock, if you aren't cooking for vegetarians.

Risotto primavera

SERVES 4–6

2 tbsp olive oil
50g (1¾oz) butter
1 onion, finely chopped
salt and freshly ground black pepper
3 garlic cloves, finely chopped
300g (10oz) arborio rice or carnaroli rice
250ml (9fl oz) white wine
600ml (1 pint) hot vegetable stock for the slow cooker (900ml/1½ pints for the traditional method)

125g (4½oz) fresh or frozen broad beans
bunch of asparagus spears, trimmed and chopped into bite-sized pieces
2 small courgettes, diced
30g (1oz) grated Parmesan cheese, plus extra for serving

in the slow cooker   **PREP** 15 MINS   **COOK** 10 MINS PRECOOKING; **AUTO/LOW** 1½–2 HRS

1 Preheat the slow cooker, if required. Heat the oil and half the butter in a large heavy-based pan over a medium heat, add the onion, and cook for 3–4 minutes until soft. Season with salt and pepper, then add the garlic and cook for a minute.

2 Stir through the rice and turn it in the oily butter so all the grains are coated. Cook for a few seconds. Increase the heat, add the wine, and let it bubble for 1–2 minutes until it has been absorbed. Transfer everything to the slow cooker, then pour in the stock and add the broad beans, asparagus, and courgettes. Cover with the lid and cook on auto/low for 1½–2 hours.

3 Stir though the remaining butter together with the Parmesan cheese, taste, and season if needed. Serve with more Parmesan and a lightly dressed wild rocket and tomato salad on the side.

traditional method   **PREP** 15 MINS   **COOK** 1 HR

1 Heat the oil and half the butter in a large heavy-based pan over a medium heat, add the onion, and cook for 3–4 minutes until soft. Season with salt and pepper, then add the garlic and cook for a minute.

2 Stir through the rice and turn it in the oily butter so all the grains are coated. Cook for a few seconds. Increase the heat, add the wine, and let it bubble for 1–2 minutes until it has been absorbed. Then add a ladleful of the hot stock at a time (keeping the rest simmering in a saucepan) and stir, cooking until it has been absorbed. Continue doing this for 30–40 minutes or until the rice is cooked to al dente and is creamy. You may not use all the stock or you may need a little more.

3 While that's cooking, add the broad beans to a large pan of boiling salted water, and cook for 3–4 minutes, then drain well and set aside. Heat the remaining oil in another frying pan over a medium heat, add the asparagus and courgettes, and cook for a few minutes until they just begin to colour. Stir all the vegetables into the risotto, dot the remaining butter all over, and stir it in. Then stir in the Parmesan cheese, taste and season, if needed. Serve with more Parmesan and a lightly dressed wild rocket and tomato salad on the side.

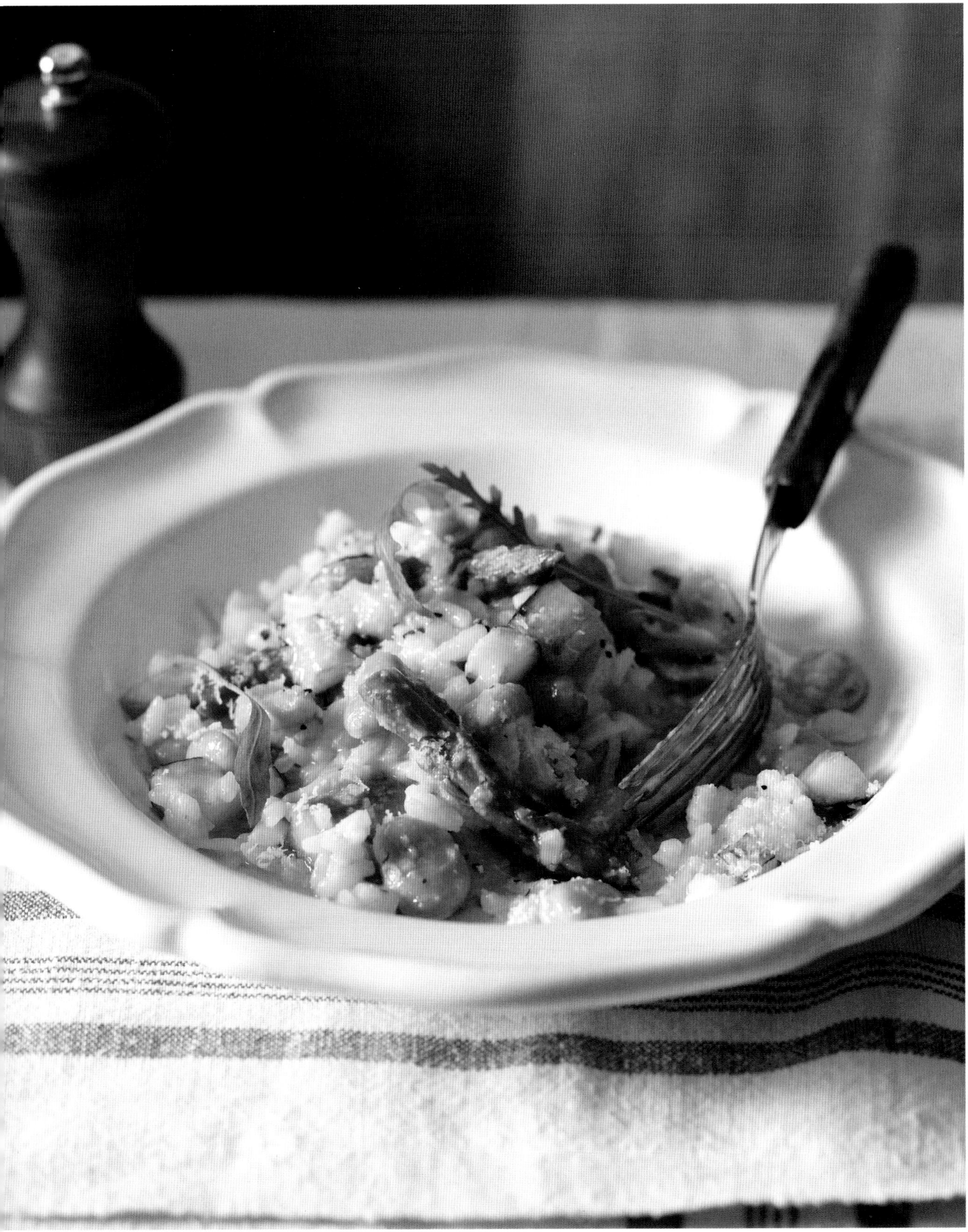

In this recipe, the rice slowly steams on top of the meat and yogurt mixture. The cardamom pods also release their aromatic flavour during the long cooking time – but don't eat them!

Saffron and lamb biryani

SERVES 4–6

1 tsp saffron threads, ground with a pestle and mortar
100ml (3½fl oz) hot milk
200g (7oz) unsalted butter
1 tsp ground cinnamon
10 cardamom pods, split
10 whole cloves
20 black peppercorns
3 bay leaves
2 large onions, diced

8 garlic cloves, peeled and chopped
1 tsp ground ginger
1 tsp ground cumin
2 tsp medium hot chilli powder
2 tsp ground coriander
350ml (12fl oz) plain yogurt
1kg (2¼lb) lean lamb, cut into bite-sized pieces
500g (1lb 2oz) easy-cook basmati rice
100g (3½oz) toasted flaked almonds

in the slow cooker

PREP 20 MINS **COOK** 15 MINS PRECOOKING;
AUTO/LOW 6–8 HRS OR **HIGH** 3–4 HRS

1 Preheat the slow cooker, if required. Put the saffron into the hot milk and set aside. Melt the butter in a large flameproof casserole, then stir in the cinnamon, cardamom, cloves, and peppercorns and cook for 5 minutes. Add the bay leaves and onions and cook for 2–3 minutes until soft.

2 Add the garlic, ginger, cumin, chilli powder, coriander, and yogurt and stir to combine, then add the lamb and half the saffron milk. Mix thoroughly and turn off the heat.

3 Bring a large pan of salted water to the boil and add the rice. Cook for about 2 minutes and drain well. Add the lamb mixture to the slow cooker and top with the rice and the remaining saffron milk. Cover with the lid and cook on auto/low for 6–8 hours or on high for 3–4 hours until the rice is tender and the lamb is cooked. Discard the cardamom pods. Stir through the toasted almonds, combine gently with a fork, and serve with chutney and chapatis.

traditional method

PREP 20 MINS **COOK** 1¾ HRS, PLUS STEAMING

1 Put the saffron into the hot milk and set aside. Melt the butter in a large flameproof casserole, then stir in the cinnamon, cardamom, cloves, and peppercorns and cook for 5 minutes. Add the bay leaves and onions and cook for 2–3 minutes until soft.

2 Add the garlic, ginger, cumin, chilli powder, coriander, and yogurt and stir to combine, then add the lamb and half the saffron milk. Mix thoroughly and turn off the heat.

3 Bring a large pan of salted water to the boil and add the rice. Cook for about 2 minutes and drain well, then tip the rice on top of the lamb mixture and pour over the remaining saffron milk. Cover the casserole tightly with foil to create a good seal, then cover it with the lid. Cook over a very low heat for 1½ hours until the rice is tender and the lamb is cooked. Check occasionally that it's not drying out, topping up with a little hot water if needed. Remove from the heat and stand for 15 minutes without opening. Uncover and discard the cardamom pods, then add the toasted almonds, combine gently with a fork, and serve with chutney and chapatis.

This delightfully simple dish is made extra tasty with a blend of parsley, thyme, and sage, which would be extra flavourful if picked freshly from the garden or pots on the windowsills.

Pork with rice and tomatoes

SERVES 4–6   **FREEZE** UP TO 3 MONTHS   **HEALTHY**

4 tbsp olive oil
2 onions, diced
900g (2lb) lean pork, cut into 5cm (2in) chunks
3 garlic cloves, finely chopped
handful of flat-leaf parsley, chopped
1 tbsp thyme leaves

1 tbsp chopped sage leaves
1 tsp paprika
150ml (5fl oz) dry white wine
225g (8oz) long-grain rice
2 x 400g cans chopped tomatoes
salt and freshly ground black pepper

in the slow cooker   **PREP** 30 MINS   **COOK** 15 MINS PRECOOKING; **AUTO/LOW** 1–1½ HRS

1 Preheat the slow cooker, if required. Heat the oil in a large flameproof casserole over a medium heat, add the onions, and cook for 4–5 minutes until soft. Add the pork and cook, stirring occasionally, for about 5 minutes until no longer pink. Add the garlic, parsley, thyme, sage, and paprika and combine, then add the wine and cook for 5 minutes. Add the rice and tomatoes, stir to combine, then season well with salt and black pepper.

2 Transfer everything to the slow cooker, cover with the lid, and cook on auto/low for 1–1½ hours. Stir halfway through, if you wish. Serve with a lightly dressed salad and crusty bread.

traditional method   **PREP** 30 MINS   **COOK** 1 HR

1 Preheat the oven to 150°C (300°F/Gas 2). Heat the oil in a large flameproof casserole over a medium heat, add the onions, and cook for 4–5 minutes until soft. Add the pork and cook, stirring occasionally, for about 5 minutes until no longer pink. Add the garlic, parsley, thyme, sage, and paprika and combine, then add the wine and cook for 5 minutes. Add the rice and tomatoes, stir to combine, then season well with salt and black pepper.

2 Cover with the lid and put in the oven for 1 hour. Check occasionally that it's not drying out, topping up with a little hot water if needed. Remove from the oven and allow to stand for 10 minutes with the lid on before serving. Serve with a lightly dressed salad and crusty bread.

Fragrant and full of colour, this pilaf has lots of layers of flavour. Swap in different dried fruits and nuts for variety. Dates and apricots are often used in Turkish dishes, as are almonds.

Turkish lamb and pomegranate pilaf

SERVES 4–6

2 tbsp olive oil, plus extra for drizzling
675g (1½lb) lamb leg, cut into bite-sized pieces
1 onion, finely chopped
salt and freshly ground black pepper
3 garlic cloves, finely chopped
1 green chilli, deseeded and finely sliced
1 tsp dried mint
1 tsp ground cinnamon
60g (2oz) golden sultanas or use regular sultanas

350g (12oz) easy-cook basmati rice
600ml (1 pint) hot lamb stock for the slow cooker
  (900ml/1½ pints for the traditional method)
60g (2oz) hazelnuts, toasted and roughly chopped
small handful of dill, finely chopped
100g (3½oz) pomegranate seeds (about 1
  pomegranate)
75g (2½oz) feta cheese, crumbled (optional)

in the slow cooker PREP 15 MINS COOK 15–20 MINS PRECOOKING; AUTO/LOW 2–3 HRS

1 Preheat the slow cooker, if required. Heat the oil in a large flameproof casserole over a medium-high heat, add the lamb (in batches, if necessary), and cook for 6–8 minutes until browned on all sides. Remove and set aside. Add the onion to the casserole and cook over a medium heat for 3–4 minutes until soft. Season with salt and pepper, stir in the garlic, chilli, mint, and cinnamon, and cook for another 2 minutes. Stir in the sultanas.

2 Stir through the rice and turn it, so all the grains are coated and the juices soaked up. Return the lamb to the casserole, pour over the stock, and bring to the boil. Transfer everything to the slow cooker, cover with the lid, and cook on auto/low for 2–3 hours, stirring halfway through, or until the rice is tender and the liquid has been absorbed. Taste and season, then stir through the hazelnuts and dill, and scatter with the pomegranate seeds. Top with crumbled feta, if using, and serve with warm pitta bread and a lightly dressed crisp green salad.

traditional method PREP 15 MINS COOK 1 HR

1 Heat the oil in a large flameproof casserole over a medium-high heat, add the lamb (in batches, if necessary) and cook for 6–8 minutes until browned on all sides. Remove and set aside.

2 Add the onion to the casserole and cook over a medium heat for 3–4 minutes until soft. Season with salt and pepper, stir in the garlic, chilli, mint, and cinnamon, and cook for another 2 minutes. Stir in the sultanas.

3 Stir through the rice and turn it, so all the grains are coated and the juices soaked up. Return the lamb to the casserole, pour over the stock, and reduce to a simmer. Partially cover and cook for 30–40 minutes, topping up with a little more hot stock if it begins to dry out. Taste and season, then stir through the hazelnuts and dill, and scatter with the pomegranate seeds. Top with crumbled feta, if using, and serve with warm pitta bread and a lightly dressed crisp green salad.

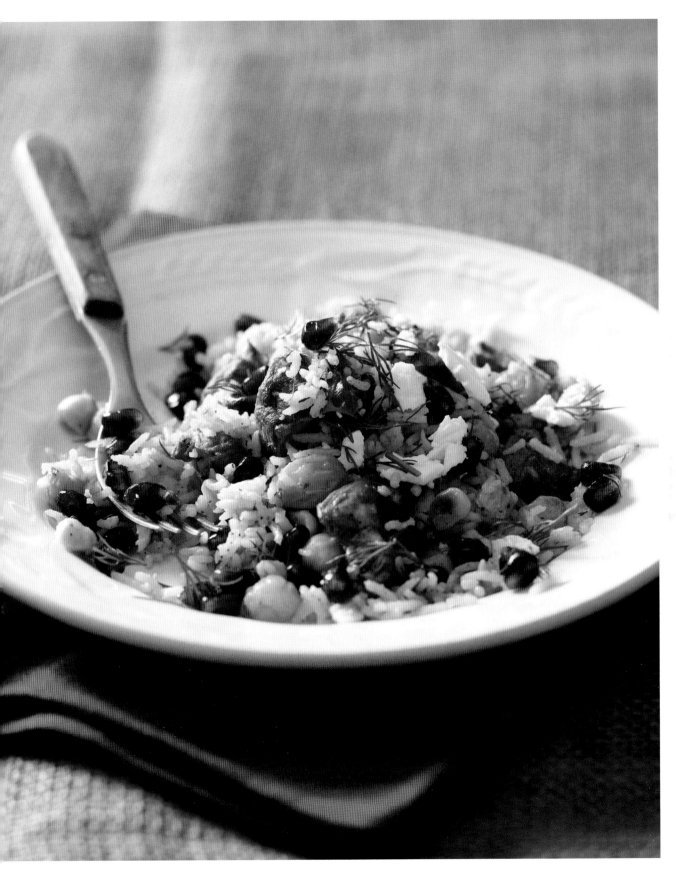

This is a traditional dish from the American South. You could cook the ham a day in advance, then chill the meat until ready to use. Dark cabbage or kale would make an ideal accompaniment.

Hoppin' John

SERVES 4–6

1 smoked ham hock, weighing about 1.1kg (2½lb)
1 bouquet garni, made with celery, thyme sprigs,
  and 1 bay leaf
2 large onions, chopped
1 dried red chilli, chopped (optional)

1 tbsp groundnut oil or sunflower oil
200g (7oz) long-grain rice
2 x 400g cans black-eyed beans, drained
  and rinsed
salt and freshly ground black pepper

in the slow cooker   **PREP** 15 MINS   **COOK** 5 MINS PRECOOKING; **AUTO/LOW** 4–6 HRS, THEN **AUTO/LOW** 2 HRS

1 Preheat the slow cooker, if required. Sit the ham hock in the slow cooker and pour in enough cold water to cover. Add the bouquet garni, half the onions, and the chilli, if using, then cover with the lid and cook on auto/low for 4–6 hours until you can pierce the ham easily with a knife. Remove the ham and set aside. Turn off the slow cooker and strain and reserve the stock. Discard the bouquet garni, onions, and chilli. Turn the slow cooker back on to auto/low.

2 Heat the oil in a heavy-based pan over a medium heat, add the remaining onion, and cook for 4–5 minutes until soft. Add the rice and stir, then transfer to the slow cooker. Add the black-eyed beans and pour over enough of the reserved stock to cover, adding a little hot water if needed. Return the ham to the slow cooker, cover with the lid, and continue cooking on auto/low for 2 hours. Stir the rice halfway through the cooking time.

3 Lift out the ham, then remove the meat from the bone and cut it into large chunks. Return the meat back to the slow cooker and stir through. Serve with steamed dark cabbage or kale and a splash of Tabasco sauce.

traditional method   **PREP** 15 MINS   **COOK** 3–3½ HRS

1 Put the ham hock in a heavy-based pan, pour in enough cold water to cover, and set over a high heat. Slowly bring to the boil, skimming the surface as necessary. Reduce the heat to low, add the bouquet garni, half the onions, and the chilli, if using, then re-cover the pan and leave to simmer for 2½–3 hours or until the meat is very tender when pierced with a knife. Remove the ham and set aside. Strain the stock and reserve.

2 Heat the oil in the pan over a medium heat, add the remaining onion, and cook for 4–5 minutes until soft. Add the rice and stir. Stir in 450ml (15fl oz) of the reserved stock and the black-eyed beans. Taste and add seasoning if needed. Bring to the boil, then reduce the heat to low, cover tightly, and simmer for 20 minutes without lifting the lid.

3 Meanwhile, remove the meat from the bone and cut it into large chunks. Remove the casserole from the heat and leave to stand for 5 minutes without lifting the lid. Using a fork, stir in the ham. Serve with steamed dark cabbage or kale and a splash of Tabasco sauce.

You could swap the chicken in this one-pot dish for ready-cooked prawns, stirring them in at the end of cooking. Apricots, dates, or figs would be worthy replacements for the sultanas.

Chicken and chickpea pilaf

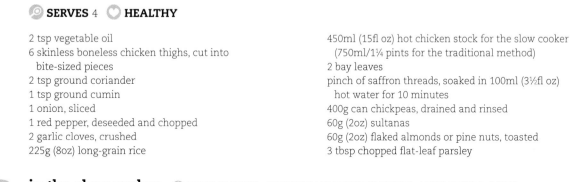

SERVES 4   **HEALTHY**

2 tsp vegetable oil
6 skinless boneless chicken thighs, cut into bite-sized pieces
2 tsp ground coriander
1 tsp ground cumin
1 onion, sliced
1 red pepper, deseeded and chopped
2 garlic cloves, crushed
225g (8oz) long-grain rice

450ml (15fl oz) hot chicken stock for the slow cooker (750ml/1¼ pints for the traditional method)
2 bay leaves
pinch of saffron threads, soaked in 100ml (3½fl oz) hot water for 10 minutes
400g can chickpeas, drained and rinsed
60g (2oz) sultanas
60g (2oz) flaked almonds or pine nuts, toasted
3 tbsp chopped flat-leaf parsley

in the slow cooker   **PREP** 20 MINS   **COOK** 20 MINS PRECOOKING; **AUTO/LOW** 2–3 HRS

1 Preheat the slow cooker, if required. Heat half the oil in a large flameproof casserole over a medium heat, add the chicken, coriander, and cumin, and cook for about 10 minutes, stirring frequently. Remove and set aside. Reduce the heat, add the rest of the oil together with the onion, red pepper, and garlic, and cook for about 10 minutes until soft.

2 Stir in the rice so all the grains are coated, then transfer everything to the slow cooker, including the chicken. Pour in the stock, or just enough to cover, and add the bay leaves and saffron with its soaking water. Stir in the chickpeas, cover with the lid, and cook on auto/low for 2–3 hours, giving it a stir halfway though. Add the sultanas for the last 30 minutes of cooking. Transfer to a warmed platter and serve hot, sprinkled with the toasted nuts and chopped parsley.

traditional method   **PREP** 20 MINS   **COOK** 45 MINS

1 Heat half the oil in a large flameproof casserole over a medium heat, add the chicken, coriander, and cumin, and cook for about 10 minutes, stirring frequently. Remove and set aside. Reduce the heat, add the rest of the oil together with the onion, red pepper, and garlic, and cook for about 10 minutes until soft.

2 Stir in the rice so all the grains are coated, return the chicken to the casserole, and pour in about three-quarters of the stock (keeping the rest simmering in a saucepan). Add the bay leaves and saffron with its soaking water, and bring to the boil. Simmer for about 20 minutes or until the rice is almost cooked, adding more stock as needed. Stir in the chickpeas and sultanas and continue cooking the pilaf on a gentle heat for about 15 minutes, stirring occasionally so it doesn't stick. Transfer to a warmed platter and serve hot, sprinkled with the toasted nuts and chopped parsley.

This light and delicately flavoured pilaf requires gentle cooking, with fresh, fragrant ingredients added just before serving. It makes a perfect summer dish – just right for outdoor dining.

Coconut, mango, and lime pilaf

SERVES 4–6

1 tbsp olive oil
1 onion, finely chopped
3 garlic cloves, finely chopped
2 red chillies, finely chopped
grated zest of 1 lime and juice of 2 limes
pinch of ground allspice
salt and freshly ground black pepper
350g (12oz) easy-cook basmati rice

60g (2oz) desiccated coconut
900ml (1½ pints) hot vegetable stock for
    the slow cooker (1.2 litres/2 pints for the
    traditional method)
1 mango, stoned, peeled, and chopped into
    bite-sized pieces
small bunch of coriander, leaves roughly chopped

in the slow cooker   **PREP** 15 MINS   **COOK** 10 MINS PRECOOKING; AUTO/LOW 2–3 HRS

1 Preheat the slow cooker, if required. Heat the oil in a large heavy-based pan over a medium heat, add the onion, and cook on a low heat for 3–4 minutes until soft. Season with salt and pepper, stir through the garlic, chillies, lime zest, and allspice, and cook for a further 2 minutes.

2 Stir through the rice, turning it until the grains are thoroughly coated, then stir through half the lime juice and the coconut. Pour in the stock, season again, and bring to the boil.

3 Transfer everything to the slow cooker, cover with the lid, cook on auto/low for 2–3 hours or until the rice is tender and the liquid has all been absorbed. Stir through the mango and coriander and add the remaining lime juice. Serve with a crisp green salad.

traditional method   **PREP** 15 MINS   **COOK** 45 MINS

1 Heat the oil in a large heavy-based pan over a medium heat, add the onion, and cook on a low heat for 3–4 minutes until soft. Season with salt and pepper, stir through the garlic, chillies, lime zest, and allspice, and cook for a further 2 minutes.

2 Stir through the rice, turning it until the grains are thoroughly coated, then stir through half the lime juice and the coconut. Pour in the stock, season again, and bring to a simmer. Partially cover with the lid and leave to cook for 30–40 minutes, stirring occasionally, and topping up with hot stock if needed. Stir through the mango and coriander and add the remaining lime juice. Serve with a crisp green salad.

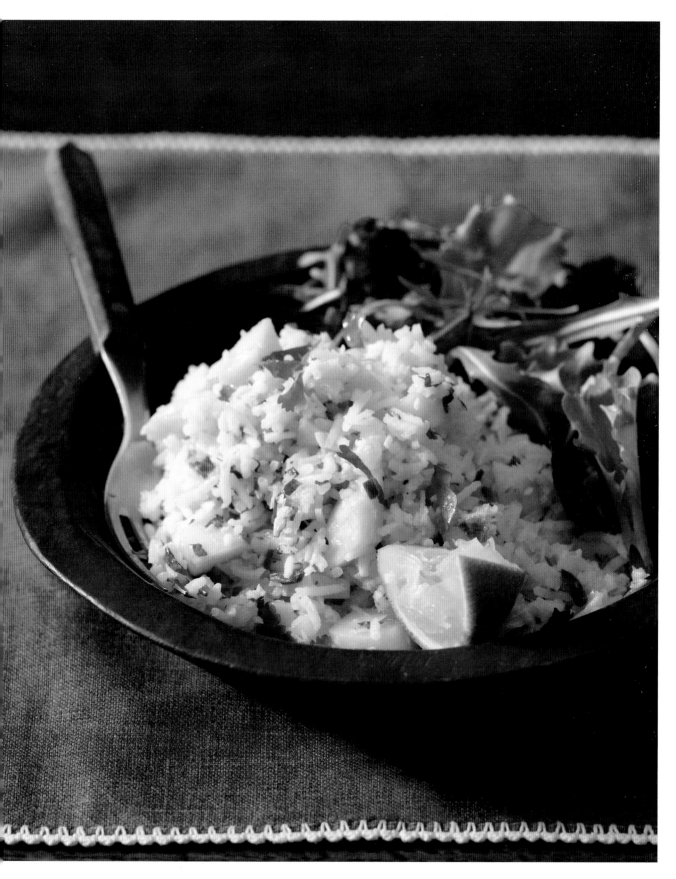

This Spanish recipe of saffron-flavoured rice with chicken, prawns, mussels, and chorizo is named after the paellera in which it is traditionally cooked. It remains a firm favourite across the world.

Paella

SERVES 4–6   **HEALTHY**

3 tbsp olive oil
400g (14oz) skinless boneless chicken thighs, cut into bite-sized pieces
salt and freshly ground black pepper
150g (5½oz) chorizo, sliced
1 large onion, diced
1 large red pepper, deseeded and sliced
400g (14oz) paella rice or other short-grain rice
3 garlic cloves, finely chopped

2 large pinches of saffron threads, soaked in 100ml (3½fl oz) hot water for 10 minutes
400g can chopped tomatoes
125g (4½oz) French beans, cut into 1cm (½in) slices
300g (10oz) small mussels, scrubbed and debearded (discard any that do not close when tapped)
300g (10oz) raw, unpeeled king prawns, deveined and legs removed
1–2 tbsp chopped flat-leaf parsley

in the slow cooker   **PREP** 20 MINS   **COOK** 20 MINS PRECOOKING; AUTO/LOW 2 HRS, THEN **HIGH** 40 MINS

1 Preheat the slow cooker, if required. Heat the oil in a wide heavy-based frying pan over a medium heat, add the chicken and seasoning, and cook for 10–12 minutes until browned all over. Remove and set aside. Cook the chorizo for 1–2 minutes on each side until browned. Also remove and set aside. Add the onion and red pepper to the pan and cook for 5–7 minutes until soft. Add the rice and stir, so all the grains are coated, and cook for 2–3 minutes. Transfer the rice to the slow cooker, add the chicken and chorizo, then add the garlic, saffron with its soaking liquid, and seasoning. Push the chicken down into the rice, add the tomatoes, and pour over 200ml (7fl oz) water, or just enough to cover.

2 Cover with the lid and cook on auto/low for 2 hours, adding the beans after 1 hour of cooking. Then turn the slow cooker to high, pour in 100ml (3½fl oz) boiling water, add the mussels and prawns, and continue cooking for 40 minutes. Remove the lid, cover with a tea towel, and let it stand for 5 minutes. Discard any mussels that haven't opened. Sprinkle with the parsley and serve.

traditional method   **PREP** 20 MINS   **COOK** 1 HR

1 Heat the oil in a wide heavy-based frying pan over a medium heat, add the chicken and seasoning, and cook for 10–12 minutes until browned all over. Remove and set aside. Cook the chorizo for 1–2 minutes on each side until browned. Also remove and set aside. Add the onion and red pepper to the pan and cook for 5–7 minutes until soft. Add the rice and stir, so all the grains are coated, and cook for 2–3 minutes. Stir in 900ml (1½ pints) water, then the garlic, saffron with its soaking liquid, and plenty of seasoning. Push the chicken pieces down into the rice. Scatter the chorizo slices over, followed by the tomatoes and beans, and bring to the boil.

2 Simmer on a low heat, uncovered, for about 30 minutes until all the liquid has evaporated and the rice is al dente. Do not stir or the rice will become sticky. If the rice is undercooked or starts to stick to the pan, add a little more hot water and simmer for a few minutes longer. Add the mussels and prawns to the pan for the last 15 minutes of cooking, cover, and cook until the mussels open and the prawns turn pink. Remove from the heat and discard any mussels that have not opened. Cover with a tea towel and let it stand for 5 minutes. Sprinkle with the parsley and serve.

Vary this colourful dish to suit your mood or your storecupboard – use chilli powder instead of paprika, or carrots instead of peas. Stir through herbs, such as parsley or coriander, at the end.

Arroz con pollo

SERVES 4   **HEALTHY**

2 tbsp olive oil
8 chicken thighs on the bone
1 Spanish onion or large onion, finely sliced
1 green pepper, deseeded and chopped
1 red pepper, deseeded and chopped
2 garlic cloves, finely chopped
1 tsp smoked paprika
1 bay leaf
200g can chopped tomatoes
1 tsp thyme leaves

1 tsp dried oregano
175g (6oz) long-grain rice
pinch of saffron threads, soaked in 100ml (3½fl oz) hot water for 10 minutes
350ml (12fl oz) hot chicken stock for the slow cooker (750ml/1¼ pints for the traditional method)
2 tbsp tomato purée
juice of ½ lemon
salt and freshly ground black pepper
100g (3½oz) frozen peas

in the slow cooker   PREP 20 MINS   COOK 20 MINS PRECOOKING; AUTO/LOW 3–3½ HRS

1 Preheat the slow cooker, if required. Heat half the oil in a large flameproof casserole over a high heat, add the chicken thighs (in batches, if necessary), and cook for about 15 minutes until browned all over. Remove and set aside.

2 Add the remaining oil, reduce the heat, and cook the onion for 4–5 minutes until soft. Add the peppers and garlic and cook for about 5 minutes until they start to soften. Add the paprika, bay leaf, tomatoes, thyme, and oregano, and stir in the rice. Fry for 1–2 minutes, stirring constantly. Transfer to the slow cooker and add the saffron with its soaking liquid, stock to cover, tomato purée, lemon juice, and seasoning.

3 Add the chicken thighs, pushing them down into the rice, cover with the lid, and cook on auto/low for 3–3½ hours. Add the peas for the last 10 minutes of cooking. Remove the bay leaf and serve hot.

traditional method   PREP 20 MINS   COOK 45 MINS

1 Preheat the oven to 180°C (350°F/Gas 4). Heat half the oil in a large flameproof casserole over a high heat, add the chicken thighs (in batches, if necessary), and cook for about 15 minutes until browned all over. Remove and set aside.

2 Add the remaining oil, reduce the heat, and cook the onion for 4–5 minutes until soft. Add the peppers and garlic and cook for about 5 minutes until they start to soften. Add the paprika, bay leaf, tomatoes, thyme, and oregano, and stir in the rice. Fry for 1–2 minutes, stirring constantly. Add the saffron with its soaking liquid, stock, tomato purée, lemon juice, and seasoning.

3 Return the chicken thighs to the casserole, pushing them down into the rice, cover with the lid, and put in the oven for 15 minutes. Add the peas and return to the oven for a further 10 minutes, or until the rice is tender and has absorbed the cooking liquid. Remove the bay leaf and serve hot.

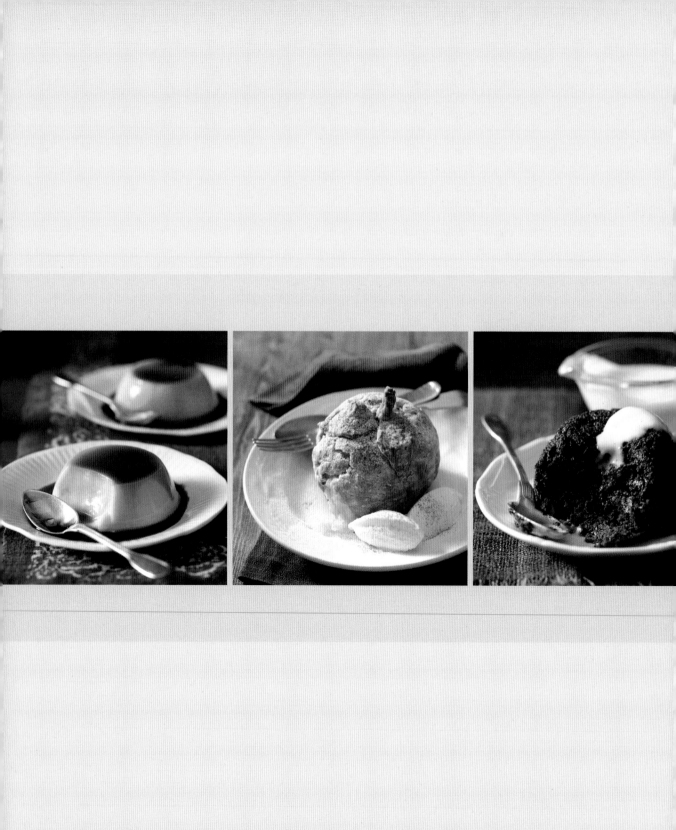

Puddings

Rich and decadent, these mini puddings are delicious served hot with some vanilla ice cream. To cook the puddings in one batch, use a slow cooker that is a minimum of 4.5 litres in size.

Chocolate and prune sponge puddings

 MAKES 6

125g (4½oz) butter, softened
125g (4½oz) caster sugar
2 eggs, beaten

125g (4½oz) self-raising flour, sifted
30g (1oz) cocoa powder, mixed with 2 tbsp milk
125g (4½oz) prunes, stoned and chopped

in the slow cooker PREP 30–40 MINS COOK HIGH 45 MINS

1 Preheat the slow cooker, if required. Grease six 150ml (5fl oz) metal pudding moulds. Put the butter and sugar into a mixing bowl and beat together until creamy and pale. Add the eggs slowly, beating as you go and adding a little flour to prevent any curdling. Then fold in the remaining flour until it is thoroughly combined, and stir through the cocoa mixture and prunes.

2 Divide the mixture between the moulds and cover each one with a pleated piece of greased greaseproof paper and a sheet of foil kept in place with string.

3 Sit the pudding moulds in the slow cooker and pour in enough boiling water to come halfway up the sides of the pudding moulds. Cover with the lid and cook on high for 45 minutes. Carefully lift the moulds out of the slow cooker, remove the string, foil, and paper, and turn out onto warmed plates. Serve hot with ice cream, cream, custard, or chocolate sauce.

traditional method PREP 30–40 MINS COOK 45 MINS

1 Grease six 150ml (5fl oz) metal pudding moulds. Put the butter and sugar into a mixing bowl and beat together until creamy and pale. Add the eggs slowly, beating as you go and adding a little flour to prevent any curdling. Then fold in the remaining flour until it is thoroughly combined, and stir through the cocoa mixture and prunes.

2 Divide the mixture between the moulds and cover each one with a pleated piece of greased greaseproof paper and a sheet of foil kept in place with string.

3 Sit the moulds in a large heavy-based pan and pour in enough boiling water to come halfway up the sides of the pudding moulds. Cover with the lid and leave to simmer gently for about 45 minutes, topping up with more boiling water as and when needed. Carefully lift the moulds out of the pan, remove the string, foil, and paper, and turn out onto warmed plates. Serve hot with ice cream, cream, custard, or chocolate sauce.

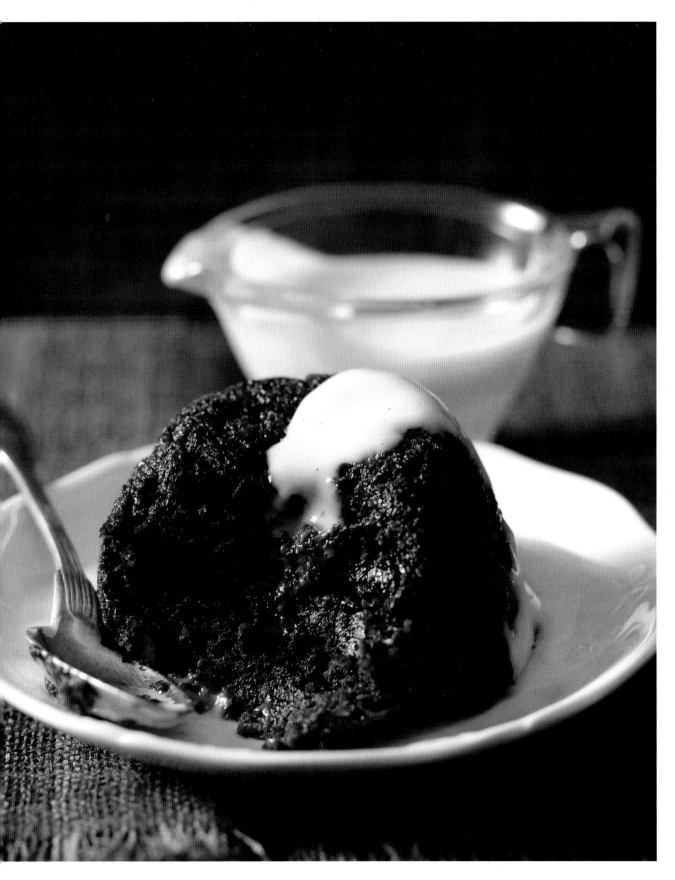

Here is a light citrussy pudding that is best enjoyed with plenty of custard. You could add a small handful of chopped almonds to the mixture for added texture.

Lemon sponge pudding

SERVES 4–6

grated zest and juice of 2 lemons
juice of ½ large orange
60g (2oz) light soft brown sugar
115g (4oz) unsalted butter, softened

60g (2oz) caster sugar
1 tbsp golden syrup
2 eggs
175g (6oz) self-raising flour, sifted

in the slow cooker **PREP** 30–40 MINS **COOK** HIGH 2–3 HRS

1 Preheat the slow cooker, if required. Grease a 1-litre (1¾-pint) pudding basin. Stir together the juice of 1 lemon with the orange juice and brown sugar in a bowl, and pour this into the pudding basin. Put the butter, caster sugar, and golden syrup into a mixing bowl along with the lemon zest and beat together until creamy and pale. Add the eggs slowly, beating as you go and adding a little flour to prevent any curdling. Then fold in the remaining flour until it is thoroughly combined and stir through the remaining lemon juice.

2 Pour the mixture into the basin and cover with a pleated piece of greased greaseproof paper and a sheet of foil. Secure with string, looping it around the basin to form a handle.

3 Sit the pudding in the slow cooker and pour in enough boiling water to come halfway up the side of the basin. Cover with the lid and cook on high for 2–3 hours. Carefully lift the basin out of the slow cooker, remove the string, foil, and paper, and turn the pudding out onto a plate. Serve piping hot with custard or cream.

traditional method **PREP** 30–40 MINS **COOK** 1½ HRS

1 Grease a 1-litre (1¾-pint) pudding basin. Stir together the juice of 1 lemon with the orange juice and brown sugar in a bowl, and pour this into the pudding basin. Put the butter, caster sugar, and golden syrup into a mixing bowl along with the lemon zest and beat together until creamy and pale. Add the eggs slowly, beating as you go and adding a little flour to prevent any curdling. Then fold in the remaining flour until it is thoroughly combined, and stir through the remaining lemon juice.

2 Pour the mixture into the basin and cover with a pleated piece of greased greaseproof paper and a sheet of foil. Secure with string, looping it around the basin to form a handle.

3 Sit the pudding bowl in a large heavy-based pan and pour in enough boiling water to come halfway up the side of the basin. Cover with the lid and leave to simmer gently for about 1½ hours, topping up with more boiling water as and when needed. Carefully lift the basin out of the pan, remove the string, foil, and paper, and turn the pudding out onto a plate. Serve piping hot with custard or cream.

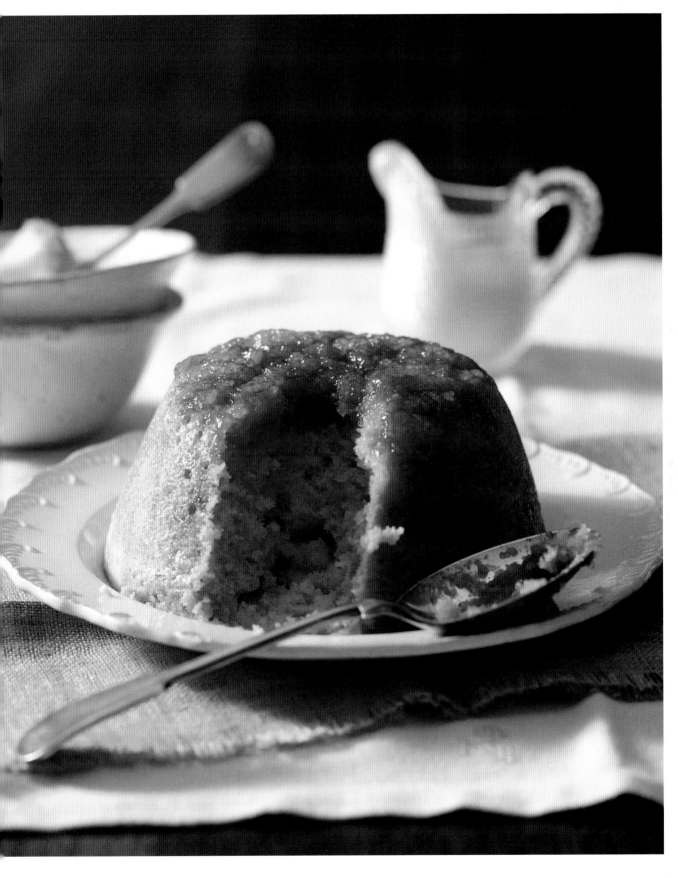

This is a delicious classic infused with the taste of vanilla. In this recipe, the seeds are discarded, but for something more aromatic, deseed the pod and add the seeds to the milk at the same time.

Classic crème caramel

 MAKES 6

600ml (1 pint) full-fat milk
1 vanilla pod, split lengthways and deseeded
225g (8oz) golden caster sugar

2 whole eggs
4 egg yolks

in the slow cooker
PREP 15 MINS, PLUS INFUSING AND CHILLING   **COOK** 25 MINS PRECOOKING; AUTO/LOW 3–4 HRS

1 Preheat the slow cooker, if required. Pour the milk into a heavy-based pan, add the vanilla pod, and very gently bring almost to the boil. Turn off the heat, cover the pan with the lid, and leave for 20 minutes. This is to give the vanilla pod time to infuse the milk while it cools.

2 Add half of the sugar to another heavy-based pan, then pour in 75ml (2½fl oz) of cold water. Slowly bring to the boil, swirling it around the pan occasionally to ensure all the sugar has dissolved, then boil for about 15 minutes, until the liquid turns a dark golden caramel. Pour this into six 150ml (5fl oz) ramekins, or use larger ones if making fewer crème caramels.

3 Put the remaining sugar with the eggs and egg yolks into a bowl and whisk until well combined and the sugar has dissolved. Discard the vanilla pod and pour the cooled milk into the egg mixture, then briefly whisk again and pour through a sieve into the ramekins. Cover each ramekin with foil and sit them in the slow cooker. Pour in enough boiling water to come halfway up the sides of the ramekins. Cover with the lid and cook on low for 3–4 hours. Lift the slow cooker dish out and leave them to cool in it, then remove the ramekins and chill them overnight in the fridge. Turn out to serve.

traditional method
PREP 15 MINS, PLUS INFUSING AND CHILLING   **COOK** 1½ HRS

1 Preheat the oven to 150°C (300°F/Gas 2). Pour the milk into a heavy-based pan, add the vanilla pod, and very gently bring almost to the boil. Turn off the heat, cover the pan with the lid, and leave for 20 minutes. This is to give the vanilla pod time to infuse the milk while it cools.

2 Add half of the sugar to another heavy-based pan, then pour in 75ml (2½fl oz) of cold water. Slowly bring to the boil, swirling it around the pan occasionally to ensure the sugar has dissolved, then boil for about 15 minutes, until the liquid turns a dark golden caramel. Pour this into six 150ml (5fl oz) ramekins, or use larger ones if making fewer crème caramels.

3 Put the remaining sugar with the eggs and egg yolks into a bowl and whisk until well combined and the sugar has dissolved. Discard the vanilla pod and pour the cooled milk into the egg mixture, then briefly whisk again and pour through a sieve into the ramekins. Sit the ramekins in a deep ovenproof dish, pour in boiling water to come two-thirds of the way up the sides of the ramekins, and cook for 1 hour. Remove the dish from the oven, leaving the ramekins in the hot water for 30 minutes to continue setting. Then leave to cool and chill overnight in the fridge. Turn out to serve.

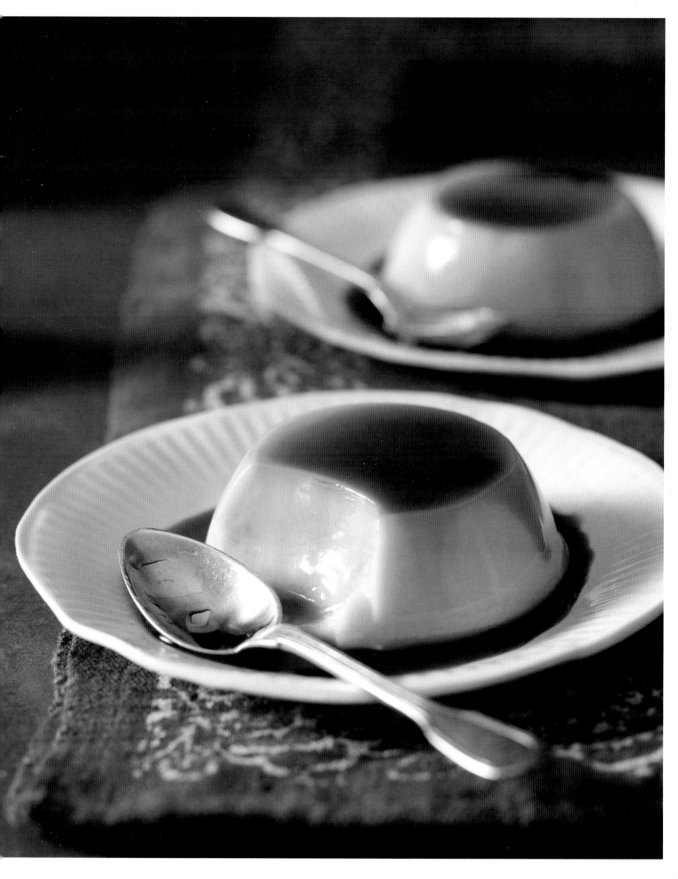

You could change the cinnamon in these dumplings for grated nutmeg or mixed spice, and use orange zest instead of lemon for a slightly sweeter finish.

Apple dumplings

SERVES 4

225g (8oz) self-raising flour, sifted
115g (4oz) vegetable suet
1 tsp ground cinnamon, plus extra to serve
grated zest of 1 lemon

4 cooking apples, peeled and cored
1 tbsp demerara sugar
60g (2oz) golden sultanas
icing sugar, to serve

in the slow cooker   PREP 20 MINS   COOK HIGH 3–4 HRS

1 Preheat the slow cooker, if required. To make the suet pastry, put the flour, suet, cinnamon, and lemon zest into a bowl. Then slowly trickle in about 100ml (3½fl oz) of cold water and mix together until it forms a dough.

2 Roll out the pastry and cut out 4 circles, large enough for each apple. Sit an apple on each round, sprinkle the demerara sugar into the apple holes, and add the sultanas to each. Brush the edges of the pastry with water and bring them together at the top, pinching to secure.

3 Turn the apples over so the sealed side is face down. If you have any pastry left over, you could fashion leaves and stalks for the dumplings. Loosely wrap foil around each and seal. Sit the dumplings in the slow cooker and add boiling water so it is about 2.5cm (1in) deep. Cover with the lid and cook on high for 3–4 hours. Lift the dumplings out of the slow cooker and remove the foil – be careful as they will be very hot. Sprinkle the dumplings with icing sugar and ground cinnamon and serve with cream, custard, or ice cream.

traditional method   PREP 20 MINS   COOK 30–40 MINS

1 Preheat the oven to 180°C (350°F/Gas 4) and lightly grease a baking sheet. To make the suet pastry, put the flour, suet, cinnamon, and lemon zest into a bowl. Then slowly trickle in about 100ml (3½fl oz) of cold water and mix together until it forms a dough.

2 Roll out the pastry and cut out 4 circles, large enough for each apple. Sit an apple on each round, sprinkle the demerara sugar into the apple holes, and add the sultanas to each. Brush the edges of the pastry with water and bring them together at the top, pinching to secure.

3 Turn the apples over so the sealed side is face down. If you have any pastry left over, you could fashion leaves and stalks for the dumplings. Sit them on the baking sheet. Cook in the oven for 30–40 minutes until golden. Sprinkle the dumplings with icing sugar and ground cinnamon and serve with cream, custard, or ice cream.

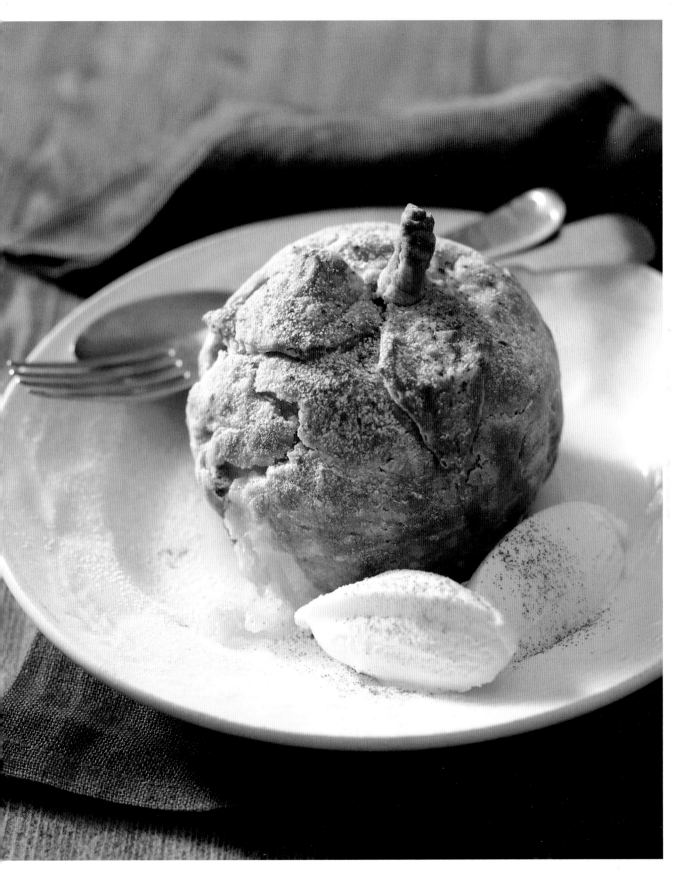

Index

Entries in *italics* indicate references to techniques.

Author

Heather Whinney is an experienced food writer and home economist. She has been the food editor of *Family Circle* and *Prima* magazines and freelance food editor at *BBC Good Food* magazine, as well as working freelance for several publications such as *Good Housekeeping* and *Woman and Home*. She is now the contributing food editor for *Prima*. As a working mother bringing up a family, she understands the issues families and busy households face when it comes to putting good food on the table. Her style and food philosophy has always remained constant – to keep it simple, and write easy recipes for the everyday cook. She is the author of *Cook Express* (2009) and co-author of *The Diabetes Cooking Book* (2010).

Acknowledgments

Heather Whinney would like to thank:

Emma Callery for excellent recipe editing and Tia Sarkar at DK for sterling hard work – what a good team we've made. Thanks to my husband Jos who is my ever-reliable recipe taster and critic and to my daughters Kim and Lorna for having healthy appetites!

Dorling Kindersley would like to thank:
Photography art direction: Luis Peral, Sara Robin
Food stylists: Katie Giovanni, Bridget Sargeson
Prop stylist: Rob Merret
Recipe testers: Jane Bamforth, Rebecca Blackstone, Louisa Carter, Sonja Edridge, Jan Fullwood, Katy Greenwood, Sylvain Jamois, Ann Reynolds, Natalie Seldon
Image retouching: Steve Crozier
Indexer: Marie Lorimer
Thanks also to Kajal Mistry, Amy Slack, and David Fentiman for editorial assistance; and to Danaya Bunnag for design assistance.